A Practical Handbook of
Joint Fluid Analysis

A Practical Handbook of Joint Fluid Analysis

Robert A. Gatter, M.D.

Physician-in-Chief
Division of Rheumatology
Abington Memorial Hospital
Abington, PA
Clinical Associate Professor of Medicine
University of Pennsylvania
Philadelphia, PA

Lea & Febiger   *1984*   *Philadelphia*

Lea & Febiger
600 Washington Square
Philadelphia, PA   19106
U.S.A.

Technical note: The "original magnifications," listed with each of the photographs of microscopic material, represent the ratio between the size of the photographic image on the original negative and the size of the microscopic specimen itself, and should be used only as an approximate indication, since they do not reflect subsequent magnifications and/or reductions in the final reproduction of the photographs.

Library of Congress Cataloging in Publication Data

Gatter, Robert A.
    A practical handbook of joint fluid analysis.

    Bibliography: p.
    Includes index.
    1. Synovia—Analysis. 2. Synovia—Examination.
3. Joints—Diseases—Diagnosis. I. Title.
RC932.G37 1983   616.7'207545   83-18704
ISBN 0-8121-0902-3

PRINTED IN THE UNITED STATES OF AMERICA

Print No.   3   2   1

To Marilyn, Anne, and Rob

Foreword

As one who has had a sustained interest in synovial fluid analysis (synovianalysis) for a quarter of a century, this practical monograph authored by a former fellow and colleague is most welcome. Robert A. Gatter, M.D., has been in the practice of clinical rheumatology for many years; his perspective relative to the performance of various tests on synovial fluid is invaluable. The material presented in the various chapters truly represents the state of the art as seen by one who daily practices that art. Most of the procedures outlined were once the province of the clinical investigator. It is heartening to those of us engaged in such investigation to see its practical application and dissemination by skilled consultants.

Rheumatology has few procedures useful in differential diagnosis relative to older disciplines such as cardiology or gastroenterology. It is particularly important, therefore, for its practitioners to know those few procedures well. It has often been stated that synovianalysis is analogous to urinalysis as the first laboratory step in the differential diagnosis of arthritis. But urine collection requires little or no skill, whereas synovial fluid collection often requires great skill in the insertion of the needle into the various joints. Obtaining a specimen is a *sine qua non* that is also addressed in this volume.

Further, this monograph represents a very useful guide for the performance and interpretation of gross, microscopic, chemical, immunologic, and microbiologic tests on such specimens. It should find a place on the bookshelf of all who wish to engage in the task of analyzing joint fluids.

Daniel J. McCarty, M.D.

Preface

The purpose of this *Handbook* is to provide a ready reference for physicians, students, and laboratory personnel interested in the study of joint fluid from the bedside to the laboratory examination, including the clinical interpretation of the results. Initially, laboratories within academic Rheumatology Divisions were the main source for providing joint fluid analysis, or synovianalysis. With the growing appreciation of the diagnostic usefulness of such analysis by primary care physicians and by medical and surgical specialists, most general hospital laboratories are, and all should be, called upon to perform it accurately. Physicians evaluating patients with arthritis may well wish to perform synovianalysis in their offices so as to have results within minutes from what is often a pathognomonic test. Medical students and house staff should find this *Handbook* an easy reference for correlation of joint fluid findings with clinical disease entities as they evaluate patients with the rheumatic diseases. Laboratory personnel without previous experience in this area should be able to initiate the technique of joint fluid analysis by following the step-by-step procedure outlined herein. The section devoted to technical notes will be helpful.

Those portions describing normal and abnormal findings, including photographs and tables to facilitate easy reference for comparing results with those in the *Handbook,* should build confidence in making accurate observations and proper interpretations. As with many laboratory procedures, joint fluid analysis provides pitfalls that mystify the beginner. Helpful hints have been included for the practical solution of these problems.

For the scientifically inquisitive, a section is included on optical crystallography as it relates to the compensated polarizing microscope. Included also are references to newer studies now being performed in research laboratories, some of which may well have future clinical application. No attempt was made to cover all of these tests or their related techniques, however, nor has there been presented an exhaustive account of all current scientific data regarding the physiology and pathology of joint fluid and the dynamic adjacent synovial lining cells.

For practical daily use, each chapter has been written in a free-standing fashion with its own reference list. Therefore, if one reads cover to cover, there will be a slight overlap in information from chapter to chapter. Basic concepts have been outlined to set the stage for our primary task: to provide a practical guide to the daily use of joint fluid analysis for the clinician and technician.

I sincerely hope that this goal has been attained and that you will be able to use this guide with comfort and confidence.

Abington, Pa.   Robert A. Gatter, M.D.

Acknowledgments

There is an old saying, "You can walk (i.e., plod) through life without friends, but you cannot run through life without them." I wish to thank those friends who helped this book do some "running."

My thanks to Daniel J. McCarty, M.D., for his foreword and his critical review of the manuscript; to Robert Irby, M.D., Paulding Phelps, M.D., Gerald P. Rodnan, M.D., and A. Dean Steele, M.D., for their critical review of the text; to George W. Campbell, Ph.D., for his review of microbiology; to H. Ralph Schumacher, M.D., for his review of the electron microscope data; and to Ronald B. Anderson, M.D., for assisting me with photography of gross and microscopic specimen.

Suzanne Schapira, who typed the entire text and tables, deserves special mention for her dedication to the project and for her helpful suggestions. Marion Chayes was most helpful in finding multiple references. John Reeder accumulated the information on microscope manufacturers, and Dorothy Rossman assisted in cataloguing many of the staining techniques found in the Appendix.

Mr. and Mrs. F. Eugene Dixon, Jr., and Mr. and Mrs. Roger L. Egleston each graciously provided sanctuary where writing could proceed uninterruptedly.

The Arthritis Foundation has kindly permitted the use of many of my own photographs and figures that had been donated to the first and second Clinical Slide Collection on the Rheumatic Diseases, Copyright 1981.

I appreciate the support of my many colleagues mentioned through these pages who provided illustrative material to complement the text.

Robert A. Gatter, M.D.

Illustrations

Color Plates

(Plates appear facing page 14.)

Tables

Contents

Chapter 1

Background

THE IMPORTANCE OF JOINT FLUID ANALYSIS

Paracelsus named joint fluid *synovia,* meaning "like egg," that is, egg *white,* which is a good way to remember that normal joint fluid is a mucinous material of high viscosity.[1] "Joint fluid" or "synovia" is correct, "synovial fluid," although a somewhat redundant term, is used frequently. Ropes and Bauer's extensive evaluation in 1953 of joint fluid in arthritic disorders divided abnormal joint fluid into two categories: Group I (noninflammatory) and Group II (inflammatory).[2] These groupings are basic and currently used terms that help compartmentalize disease entities. Subsequently, Group III (infectious disorders) was separated from the original Group II,[3] and later, the hemorrhagic group was removed from the original Group I,[4] to further highlight their clinical importance.

Joint fluid analysis was called "synovianalysis" by Dr. Joseph L. Hollander and his associates in 1961.[5] This test was and is as important to the evaluation of joint disease as urinalysis is to the detection of renal disease.[3] The truth of this analogy was most pertinent at that time, as it coincided with the recognition that monosodium urate monohydrate (MSUM) crystals were present in the joint fluid from patients with acute gout.[6] Shortly thereafter, McCarty and co-workers discovered that calcium pyrophosphate dihydrate (CPPD) crystals were present in joint fluid of patients with acute gout-like attacks called "pseudogout."[7] The subsequent

1

documentation of these facts produced a great impetus for the evaluation of joint fluid by the clinician as the most simple, rapid, and pathognomonic test in the study of arthritic disorders.

When synovial fluid white blood cell peripheral cytoplasmic inclusion bodies (CIB) were reported,[8] documented,[9] and demonstrated to contain immunoglobulins,[10,11] research rheumatologists and immunologists also focused attention on synovia.

Currently, synovianalysis is firmly established in the clinical evaluation of joint disease. Its importance is such that a careful search for even small joint effusions should be performed routinely on all patients with joint disease. Such care will provide greater opportunity for aspiration and will subsequently increase diagnostic information. Recent information indicates that even asymptomatic first metatarsal phalangeal joints, when aspirated, may confirm the presence of MSUM and CPPD crystals in patients with gout and pseudogout, respectively.[12,13]

Today, "routine synovianalysis" is generally meant to include a gross evaluation for volume, viscosity, color, and clarity, plus a microscopic examination including a total white blood cell (WBC) count, a differential WBC count, especially polymorphonuclear leukocytes (PMN), lymphocytes, monocytes, macrophages, and synoviocytes, and evaluation of a wet preparation for crystals and other pathologic material by compensated polarized light microscopy. In addition, many other studies can be performed on synovia, as detailed in the upcoming chapters.

The purpose of analyzing joint fluid is to determine the diagnosis of a given form of arthritis. The use of gross criteria will allow one to place a fluid into one of the following categories: noninflammatory, inflammatory, septic, and hemorrhagic. Each of these groups relates to a series of specific disease entities (see Tables 1-1 and 1-2). Once the type of disorder is defined, the most appropriate treatment can begin. Gout, pseudogout, other crystal deposition diseases, and septic joints can be diagnosed through joint fluid findings alone. The fact that these disorders are exquisitely painful (and, in the case of septic arthritis, rapidly destructive) yet eminently treatable only makes it more imperative that joint fluid examinations be used to the fullest extent possible.

PHYSIOLOGY AND PATHOPHYSIOLOGY OF JOINT FLUID

A joint develops embryonically as a tissue space without a limiting membrane. Several layers of specially adapted synovial cells (synoviocytes) line the joint cavity. These cells of the synovium secrete hyaluronate, a high-molecular-weight glycosaminoglycan that, by its long-branching physical configuration, tends to increase viscosity of synovia.[14] The rest of the constituents of synovia are derived from plasma as a dialysate from the capillary bed subjacent to the synovium.[15] Notable exceptions in normal joint fluid are the absence of prothrombin, fibrinogen, factor V, factor VII, tissue thromboplastin, antithrombin, larger globulins, and some components of complement.[16] This protein dysequilibrium probably is a function of the endothelial lining of the microvascular circulation. Normal fluid does not clot. If normal barriers are altered by inflammation, however, larger molecules can enter the joint fluid, and clotting can occur. In rheumatoid arthritis, local production of immunoglobulins is an additional source of specific proteins.[17,18] As permeability into the joint space increases, of course, joint fluid volume increases. Therefore, the findings expected in inflammation would be somewhat different from normal, with an increased amount of proteins and some different proteins, in addition to the changes noted in Table 1–1.

For those interested in the current concepts of the causes for joint inflammation as mediated through immunologic and crystalline stimuli, standard texts of rheumatology will provide much information and many references.[19,20]

REFERENCES

1. Field, E.J., and Harrison, R.J.: *Anatomical Terms: Their Origin and Derivation.* 2nd Edition, Cambridge-Heffer, 1957.
2. Ropes, M.W., and Bauer, W.: *Synovial Fluid Changes in Joint Disease.* Cambridge, Harvard University Press, 1953.
3. Coggeshall, H.C., in *Arthritis and Allied Conditions.* 6th Edition. Edited by J.L. Hollander. Philadelphia, Lea & Febiger, 1960.
4. Gatter, R.A., and McCarty, D.J.: Synovianalysis, a rapid clinical diagnostic procedure. Rheumatism, 20:2–6, 1964.
5. Hollander, J.L., Jessar, R.A., and McCarty, D.J.: Synovianalysis: An aid in arthritis diagnosis. Bull. Rheum. Dis., 12:263-264, 1961.
6. McCarty, D.J., and Hollander, J.L.: Identification of urate crystals in gouty synovial fluid. Ann. Intern. Med., 54:452, 1961.
7. McCarty, D.J., Kohn, N.N., and Faires, J.S.: The significance of calcium phosphate crystals in the synovial fluid of arthritis patients: The "pseudogout syndrome." I. Clinical Aspects. Ann. Intern. Med., 56:711, 1962.
8. Gatter, R.A., and McCarty, D.J., in Pseudogout syndrome. V. A clinical analysis of 30 cases. Presented at American Rheumatism Association Annual Scientific Session, Atlantic City, June, 1963.
9. Hollander, J.L., McCarty, D.J., Astorga, G., and Castro-Murillo, C.:

Table 1–1. *Joint Fluid Characteristics*

	Normal	GROUP I (Noninflammatory)	GROUP II (Inflammatory)	GROUP III (Septic)
Volume (knee, in ml)	<3.5	<3.5	>3.5	>3.5
Viscosity	Very high	High*	Low	Variable
Color	Clear	Xanthrochromic	Xanthrochromic to opalescent	Variable with organisms
Clarity	Transparent	Transparent	Translucent, opaque at times	Opaque
Mucin clot	Firm	Firm	Friable	Friable
WBC/mm³	200	200–2,000	2,000–100,000	>50,000† usually >100,000
PMN (%)	<25	<25	>50	>75†
Culture	Negative	Negative	Negative	Usually positive

*Rapid accumulation of fluid will lower viscosity.
†May be lower with partially treated or low-virulence organism.

Table 1–2. *Differential Diagnoses by Joint Fluid Groups**

GROUP I (Noninflammatory)	GROUP II (Inflammatory)	GROUP III (Septic)	GROUP IV (Hemorrhagic)
Osteoarthritis	Rheumatoid disease	Bacterial infections	Trauma with or without fracture
Traumatic arthritis	Crystal-induced synovitis		Charcot's arthropathy
Avascular necrosis	gout		Hemorrhagic diathesis
Internal derangement	pseudogout		anticoagulant therapy
Osteochondritis dissecans	hydroxyapatite		von Willebrand's
Osteochondromatosis	corticosteroid injection		Hemophilia
Charcot's arthropathy	Psoriatic arthritis		Scurvy
Subsiding inflammation	Reactive arthritis		Thrombocytopenia
Villonodular synovitis	Reiter's syndrome		Hemangioma
Hypertrophic pulmonary osteoar-thropathy	Regional enteritis		Tumor
Systemic lupus erythematosus†	Ulcerative colitis		pigmented villonodular synovitis
	Postileal bypass		synovioma

Rheumatic fever†
Scleroderma†
Amyloidosis†
Myxedema
Acromegaly
Hemochromatosis
Gaucher's disease
Ochronosis
Paget's disease of bone
Sickle cell disease

Yersinia
Campylobactor
Whipple's disease
Connective tissue disease
Systemic lupus
Polyarteritis
Scleroderma
Polymyositis
Vasculitis (nonspecific)
Polymyalgia rheumatica
Polychondritis
Sarcoidosis
Behçet's syndrome
Ankylosing spondylitis
Juvenile rheumatoid arthritis
Rheumatic fever
Agammaglobulinemia
Infectious arthritis
  (low-virulence)
  viral
  fungal
  bacterial
  mycobacterial
  mycoplasmal
Hypersensitivity
  serum sickness
  erythema multiform

*Partial listing.
†May be Group I or II.

Studies on the pathogenesis of rheumatoid joint inflammation. I. The "R.A." cell and a working hypothesis. Ann. Intern. Med., *62*:271, 1965.

10. Rawson, A.J., Abelson, N.M., and Hollander, J.L.: Studies on the pathogenesis of rheumatoid joint inflammation. Ann. Intern. Med., *62*:281, 1965.

11. Brandt, K., Cathcart, E.S., and Cohen, A.J.: Studies of immune deposits in synovial membranes and corresponding synovial fluid. J. Lab. Clin. Med., *72*:631, 1968.

12. Weinberg, A., Schumacher, H.R., and Agudelo, C.A.: Urate crystals in asymptomatic metatarsal phalangeal joints. Ann. Intern. Med., *91*:56, 1979.

13. Dorwart, B.B.: Pseudogout crystals in asymptomatic toe joints. Presented at American Rheumatism Association, Southeastern meeting, Charleston, S.C., December, 1980.

14. Ogston, A.G., and Phelps, C.F.: The partition of solutes between buffer solutions and solutions containing hyaluronate. Biochem. J., *78*:827, 1961.

15. Ropes, M.W., Rossmeisl, E.C., and Bauer, W.: The origin and nature of normal synovial fluid. J. Clin. Invest., *19*:795, 1940.

16. Cho, M.H., and Neuhaus, O.W.: Absence of blood clotting substances from synovial fluid. Thromb. Diath. Haemorrh., *5*:108, 1960.

17. Kushner, I., and Somerville, J.: Permeability of human synovial membrane to plasma protein. Arthritis Rheum., *14*:560, 1971.

18. Pruzanski, W., et al.: Serum and synovial fluid proteins in rheumatoid arthritis and degenerative joint disease. Am. J. Med. Sci., *265*:483, 1973.

19. Fearson, D.T., and Auslen, K.F.: Acute inflammatory response. In *Arthritis and Allied Conditions.* Edited by D.J. McCarty. Philadelphia, Lea & Febiger, 1979.

20. W.A. Kelley, et al. (Eds.): *Textbook of Rheumatology.* Philadelphia, W.B. Saunders, 1981, Chapters 1-13, 58, 59.

Chapter 2

Joint Aspiration: Indications and Technique

INDICATIONS

Joint fluid aspiration is diagnostically indicated in any patient with an effusion who has an undiagnosed arthritic disorder or who has a new event relating to the joint with the effusion. Aspiration of inflamed, localized, periarticular soft tissue also is indicated. Even asymptomatic metatarsophalangeal joints with no evidence of active arthritis have been aspirated and found to contain MSUM and CPPD crystals.[1,2] In skilled hands, the discomfort and the risk are minimal. Therefore, in view of the valuable diagnostic information to be obtained, "DO NOT WAIT; ASPIRATE."

DETECTION OF EFFUSIONS

Detecting joint effusions requires practice. Knee joint effusions are common and easiest to discover. Once these effusions can be demonstrated with confidence, other joint effusions will become more apparent. Hip and shoulder effusions, however, are difficult to appreciate until they are quite large.

To examine the knee for an effusion, place the patient in the supine position. Note the medial aspect of the knee; a concavity is normally present posterior to (below) the medial patellar margin. If this concavity is not present, an effusion is quite likely to be

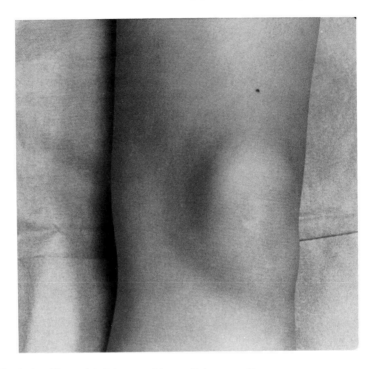

Fig. 2–1. Normal left knee with medial concavity.

present. To demonstrate the commonly found moderate or small knee effusion requires the presence of a positive "bulge" sign. The extremity should be externally rotated 30° to 45°. This should be a position of comfort, although at times it is not because of limited motion of the hip joint, and the position will have to be modified. Assuming the optimal position, use both hands to milk the fluid from the medial aspect of the joint space toward the dependent lateral side of the joint space. Then, using the thumbs of both hands placed posterior to (below), not on, the lateral margin of the patella, press the anticipated fluid back toward the medial aspect. Observe the medial concavity for the appearance of a slightly delayed bulge, known commonly as a positive "bulge sign" (Figs. 2–1, 2–2, 2–3, and 2–4).[3] The accidental medial movement of the patella should not be confused with a positive "bulge." Patellar movement would be immediate and should not be delayed, as with the fluid wave. When synovial thickening or excessive adipose tissue is present, evaluation of effusions is more difficult. A large effusion may be difficult to demonstrate, because the joint is too tense to have a bulge sign. Tapping over the patella may produce a "click" as the

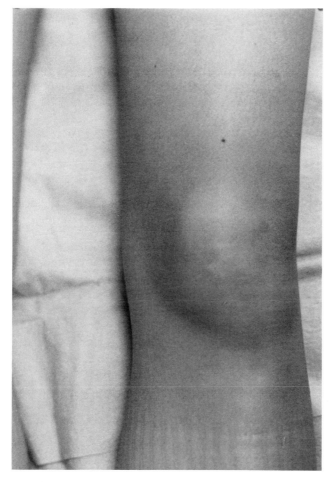

Fig. 2–2.   Left knee effusion with medial convexity.

floating patella contacts the underlying femur. This form of bal-
lottement is not reliable in all cases. Therefore, when in doubt,
remember the motto: "DO NOT WAIT; ASPIRATE."

TECHNIQUE

The technique of joint fluid aspiration (arthrocentesis) for each
type of joint has been presented in many booklets and texts, which
are easily obtainable.[4,5] Therefore, only the general principles,
using the knee as a model, will be described here.

For a large effusion, a lateral approach directly into the center

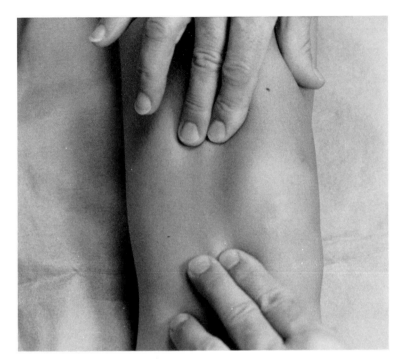

Fig. 2–3. Milking the fluid medially to laterally.

of the ballooned-out suprapatellar pouch is swift and hence less uncomfortable. The ballooning of the suprapatellar pouch can be accentuated by pressure laterally on the medial aspect of this area. With the tip of a ballpoint pen (writing point retracted), mark the target area, which will be approximately at the level of the cephalad border of the patella. This will leave a small round skin indentation sufficiently visible to allow time for cleansing, anesthesia, and arthrocentesis (Fig. 2-5).

A medial approach under the midpoint of the patella is preferable for small effusions. Be sure to allow an extra 1 to 2 centimeters posterior to the medial edge of the patella so as not to strike its "V-shaped" gliding surface (Fig. 2–6).

A word of caution about septic contamination of a sterile joint is necessary. Joint infection caused by carrying skin bacteria into the joint via the aspirating needle is rare with currently used disposable equipment and proper sterile technique. Great caution must be taken, however, not to aspirate a sterile joint in a patient with bacteremia or in one who has cutaneous or extra-articular soft tissue infection masquerading as an acute arthritis. These latter two

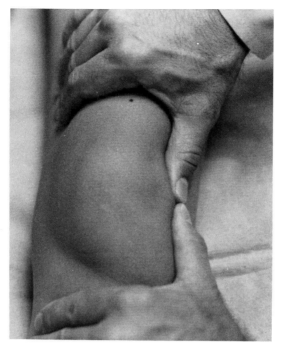

Fig. 2–4. A positive "bulge" sign appears medially.

Table 2–1. *Arthrocentesis Tray*

Syringes of choice
Needles
    25-gauge for small joints
    21-gauge for other joints
    15- to 18-gauge for thick effusions (pus, rice bodies)
Iodine disinfectant (Betadine)
Alcohol
Sterile sponges
Ethyl chloride spray
Forceps (hemostat)
Ballpoint pen with retractable point
Adhesive bandages (Band-Aid)
Clear glass, stoppered test tube with anticoagulant (sodium heparin or EDTA)
Screw-top sterile culture tube
Special items of choice
    chemistry tubes
    culture medium
    intra-articular corticosteroids

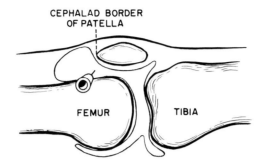

Fig. 2–5. Arthrocentesis of the right knee, lateral approach to the supra-patellar pouch.

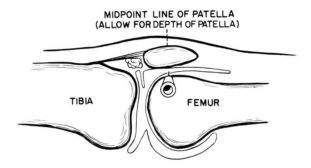

Fig. 2–6. Arthrocentesis of the right knee, medial approach under the patella.

circumstances are the likely causes of most iatrogenic septic joints. Otherwise, using strict sterile technique, there is no need for sterile gloves and drapes when performing an arthrocentesis. Proper cleansing of the skin is performed by swabbing with alcohol to remove natural oils and debris followed by an iodine-based anti-septic, such as povidone-iodine (Betadine), followed by alcohol swabbing (Table 2-1).

Spraying the designated area with ethyl chloride, which is sterile, decreases superficial pain. Do not swirl the spray, hold it steady, and stop spraying as soon as the first sign of freezing occurs; skin damage can occur in patients with atrophic skin. A quick, decisive thrust through the skin with a disposable 21-gauge needle and attached syringe produces the least discomfort. Once into the sub-cutaneous tissue, where nerve endings are less prevalent, angles and landmarks can be briefly re-evaluated so that a second pene-tration may be made through the capsule, the other area of in-creased pain fibers. This second thrust is made more cautiously because of the subjacent bone and articular cartilage. If the per-iosteum is struck, pain is considerable; if the articular cartilage is entered, a gouge may occur that does not readily heal. Therefore, it is important to pierce the capsule and enter the joint space cleanly without glancing off other structures. Small knee effusions may be withdrawn more easily if gentle pressure is applied to the opposite side of the joint cavity, bringing the fluid toward the needle tip. Once sufficient fluid has been drawn into the syringe, tension on the plunger should be released and the needle quickly withdrawn. If, during arthrocentesis, extraneous blood begins to invade the synovia in the syringe, it is usually wise to terminate the procedure to avoid excessive contamination of the fluid with blood.

At times, it is difficult to aspirate fluid in spite of its presence. In the case of chronic inflammatory arthritis, small bits (biopsies) are often aspirated if the needle touches the synovium; likewise, free-floating "rice bodies," made up of synovial tissue and/or fibrin, can clog the needle. The choices are: (1) to withdraw the needle with tissue worthy of examination in the bore, if sufficient fluid for examination is in the syringe; (2) to leave the needle in place, express some of the aspirated synovia back through the needle to unplug it, and continue with further aspiration; or (3) if neither approach has been productive, to withdraw and re-enter the joint with a larger-gauge needle.

A note of caution: it is wise to have a small surgical forceps (hemostat) with you during all aspirations and injections. Rarely, the needle may break or separate from its plastic adapter, requiring immediate retrieval from the injection site. Commonly, the forceps is useful for removing the needle from the syringe smoothly when switching syringes with the needle in the joint cavity, for example, upon aspiration and subsequent injection.

REFERENCES

1. Weinberg, A., Schumacher, H.R., and Agudelo, C.A.: Urate crystals in asymptomatic metatarsal phalangeal joints. Ann. Intern. Med., 91:56, 1979.
2. Dorwart, B.B.: Pseudogout crystals in asymptomatic toe joints. Pre-

sented, American Rheumatism Association, Southeastern meeting, Charleston, SC, December, 1980.
3. Hunder, G.G., and Polley, H.F.: Detecting small effusions of the knee. Postgrad. Med., *40*:689, 1966.
4. Pruce, A.M., Miller, J.A., and Berger, I.R.: Anatomic landmarks in joint paracentesis. Clin. Symp., *10*:3, 1958.
5. Hollander, J.L.: Arthrocentesis and intrasynovial therapy. In *Arthritis and Allied Conditions*. 9th Edition. Philadelphia, Lea & Febiger, 1979.

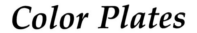

Color Plates

Plate 1.

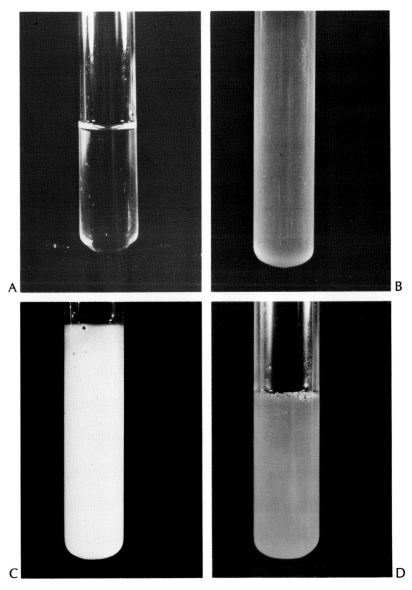

Color: *A*, Normal; *B*, Group I (noninflammatory) and Group II (inflammatory); *C*, Group III (septic); *D*, Group IV (hemorrhagic).

Plate 2.

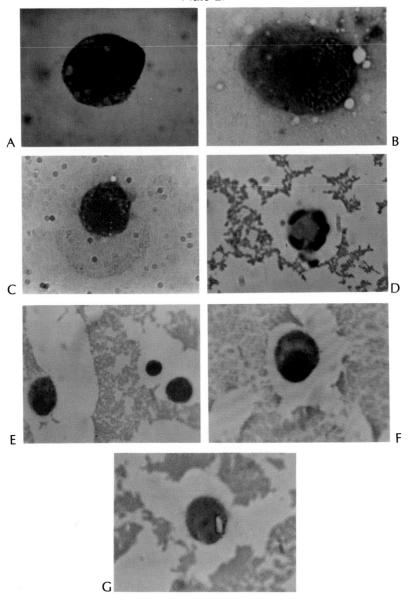

A, Synovial lining cells, phagocytic, Type A. Note vacuolated cytoplasm and nucleus:cytoplasm ratio of less than 1. Wright's stain B, Synovial lining cells, synthetic, Type B. Note homogeneous cytoplasm and nucleus:cytoplasm ratio of less than 1. Wright's stain (*A* and *B* from Schumacher, H.R.: Synovial fluid analysis. In *Textbook of Rheumatology*. Edited by William Kelley. Philadelphia, W.B. Saunders, 1981.) *C*, Monocyte (Sudan Black). Note nucleus:cytoplasm ratio is greater than 1. (Courtesy of H. Ralph Schumacher.) *D*, LE cell in joint fluid. Wright's stain (×1250). *E*, Large (stimulated) lymphocyte, small lymphocyte, medium lymphocyte (left to right). Wright's stain (×1250). *F*, Plasma cell. Wright's stain (×1250). (*E* and *F* from Gatter, R.A., and Richmond, J.D.: Predominance of synovial fluid lymphocytes in early rheumatoid arthritis. J. Rheumatol., 2:340, 1975.) *G*, Calcium pyrophosphate crystal within white blood cell. Wright's stain (×1250).

Plate 3.

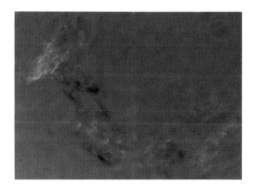

Sheaves of monosodium urate monohydrate crystals in renal parenchyma; biopsy, unstained frozen section, compensated polarized light (× 480). (From Gatter, R.A.: Use of the compensated polarizing microscope, In *Crystal Induced Arthropathies*. Edited by William N. Kelley. Clinics in Rheumatic Diseases. Vol. 3. London, W.B. Saunders, 1977.)

All crystals are photographed so that the position of the orienting (length slow) line of the compensator is from the lower left to the upper right of each page, as indicated (arrow) in Plates 4 and 5.

Plate 4.

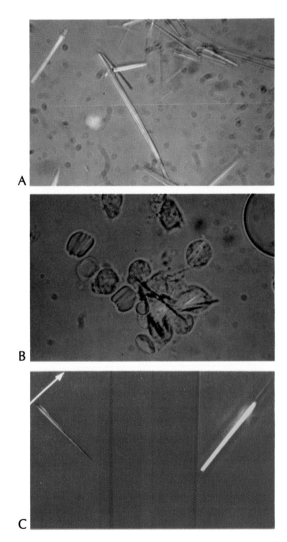

A, Monosodium urate monohydrate crystals, extracellular. Compensated polarized light (× 1250).
B, Monosodium urate monohydrate crystals, intracellular. Compensated polarized light (× 1250).
C, Monosodium urate monohydrate crystal rotated through 90°, note the color change and extinction in the plane of the polarizer. Compensated polarized light (× 1250). White arrow indicates the length slow (γ) orientation of the compensator.

All crystals are photographed so that the position of the orienting (length slow) line of the compensator is from the lower left to the upper right of each page, as indicated (arrow) in Plates 4 and 5.

Plate 5.

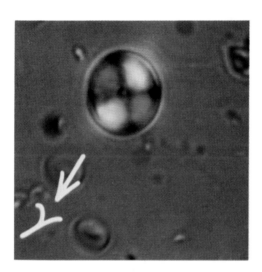

Monosodium urate monohydrate spherule; made up of many needle-shaped crystals each with one end at the center and the other at the surface, thus exhibiting typical negative elongation for each internal crystal. Compensated polarized light ($\times$ 1000). White arrow indicates the length slow (γ) orientation of the compensator. (From Fiechtner, J.J., and Simkin, P.A.: Urate spherulites in gouty synovia. JAMA, *245*:1533, 1981.)

All crystals are photographed so that the position of the orienting (length slow) line of the compensator is from the lower left to the upper right of each page, as indicated (arrow) in Plates 4 and 5.

Plate 6.

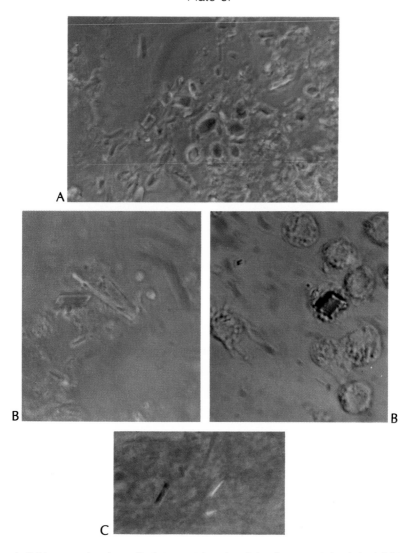

A, Calcium pyrophosphate dihydrate crystals, extracellular. Compensated polarized light (×1250). (From Gatter, R.A.: Use of the compensated polarizing microscope. In *Crystal Induced Arthropathies.* Edited by William Kelley. Clinics in Rheumatic Diseases. Vol. 3. London, W.B. Saunders, 1977.) *B,* Calcium pyrophosphate dihydrate crystals, intracellular. Compensated polarized light (×1250). *C,* Calcium pyrophosphate and urate crystals in the same joint fluid. Compensated polarized light (×1250).

All crystals are photographed so that the position of the orienting (length slow) line of the compensator is from the lower left to the upper right of each page, as indicated (arrow) in Plates 4 and 5.

Plate 7.

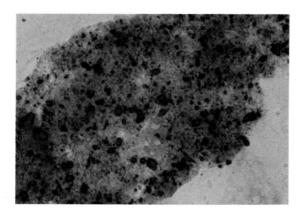

Alizarin red S stain is positive for calcium. Shown here are clumps of hydroxyapatite crystals in a joint fluid clot (ordinary light, original magnification ×100). (From Paul, H., Reginato, A.J., and Schumacher, H.R.: Alizarin red S staining as a screening test to detect calcium compounds in synovial fluid. Arthritis Rheum., 26:191, 1983.)

Plate 8.

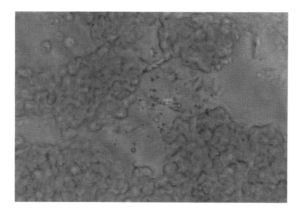

Calcium hydrogen phosphate dihydrate (Brushite). Compensated polarized light (×1250). (From Utsinger, P.D.: Dicalcium phosphate deposition disease; a suspected new crystal-induced arthritis. Presented XIV International Congress of Rheumatology. San Francisco, June, 1977.)

All crystals are photographed so that the position of the orienting (length slow) line of the compensator is from the lower left to the upper right of each page, as indicated (arrow) in Plates 4 and 5.

Plate 9.

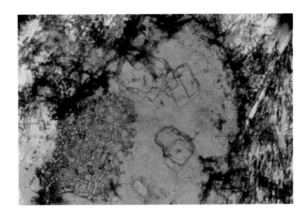

Cholesterol crystals, multiple. Note notched corners. Compensated polarized light (×100).

All crystals are photographed so that the position of the orienting (length slow) line of the compensator is from the lower left to the upper right of each page, as indicated (arrow) in Plates 4 and 5.

Plate 10.

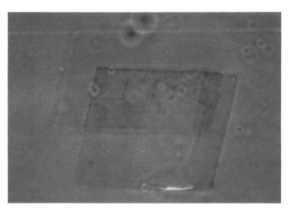

Cholesterol crystals: A few overlying one another. Note regular corners but irregular stacking stimulating notched corners. Compensated polarized light (×1250). (From Gatter, R.A.: Use of the compensated polarizing microscope. In *Crystal Induced Arthropathies*. Edited by William Kelley. Clinics in Rheumatic Diseases. Vol. 3. London, W.B. Saunders, 1977.)

All crystals are photographed so that the position of the orienting (length slow) line of the compensator is from the lower left to the upper right of each page, as indicated (arrow) in Plates 4 and 5.

Plate 11.

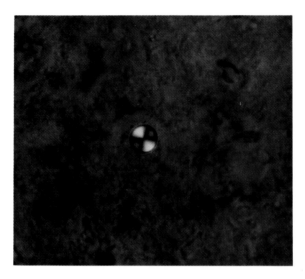

Lipid liquid crystal. Compensated polarized light (×60). (From Reginato, A.J., Schumacher, H.R., Allan, D., and Rabinowitz, J.L.: Acute monoarthritis associated with lipid liquid crystals. Arthritis Rheum., 25:535, 1982; Abstract.)

All crystals are photographed so that the position of the orienting (length slow) line of the compensator is from the lower left to the upper right of each page, as indicated (arrow) in Plates 4 and 5.

Plate 12.

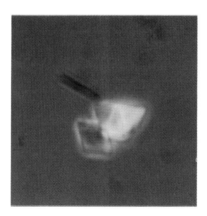

Calcium oxalate crystals. Compensated polarized light (×1250). (From Gatter, R.A.: Use of the compensated polarizing microscope. In *Crystal Induced Arthropathies*. Edited by William Kelley. Clinics in Rheumatic Diseases. Vol. 3. London, W.B. Saunders, 1977.)

All crystals are photographed so that the position of the orienting (length slow) line of the compensator is from the lower left to the upper right of each page, as indicated (arrow) in Plates 4 and 5.

Plate 13.

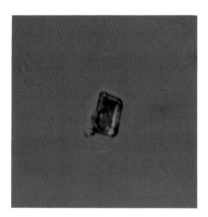

Lithium heparin crystal artifact in synovial fluid. Compensated polarized light (×1000). (From Tanphaichitr, K., Spilberg, I., and Hahn, B.H.: Lithium crystals simulating calcium pyrophosphate dihydrate crystals in synovial fluid. Arthritis Rheum., *19*:966, 1976.)

All crystals are photographed so that the position of the orienting (length slow) line of the compensator is from the lower left to the upper right of each page, as indicated (arrow) in Plates 4 and 5.

Plate 14.

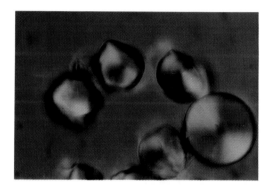

Talc crystals showing maltese cross. Compensated polarized light ($\times$1250).

All crystals are photographed so that the position of the orienting (length slow) line of the compensator is from the lower left to the upper right of each page, as indicated (arrow) in Plates 4 and 5.

Plate 15.

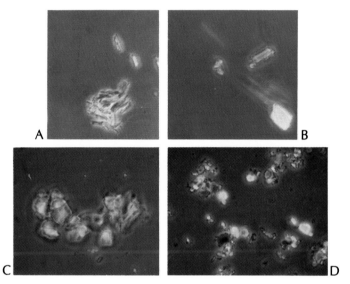

A, Prednisolone tebutate (Hydeltra-T.B.A.). Compensated polarized light (×1250). B, Triamcinolone hexacetonide (Aristospan). Compensated polarized light (×1250). C, Triamcinolone ace-
tonide (Kenalog). Compensated polarized light (×1250). D, Methylprednisolone acetate (Depo-
Medrol). Compensated polarized light (×1250).

All crystals are photographed so that the position of the orienting (length slow) line of the compensator is from the lower left to the upper right of each page, as indicated (arrow) in Plates 4
and 5.

Plate 16.

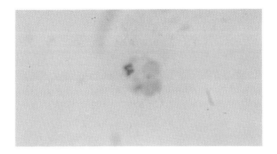

Staphylococci within leukocyte. Gram stain (× 1000).

Chapter 3

Gross Synovianalysis at the Bedside

With this technique, arthritis can be categorized accurately as noninflammatory, inflammatory, possibly septic, or hemorrhagic.

VOLUME

Although exact volumes of synovia aspirated have no diagnostic value, approximations are useful. Serial determinations reflect changes in intensity of local irritation, inflammation, or infection. Synovia is found in every joint with a synovial lining. A normal knee joint contains up to 4 ml of synovia. Since it is impossible to aspirate all of it, an aspirated volume of greater than 3.5 ml would be an abnormal accumulation. Therefore, aspirated volumes should be recorded at the bedside prior to sending the fluid to the various laboratory areas (see Table 1-1).

VISCOSITY

Having removed the needle from the syringe, express the synovia one drop at a time. Note the stringing effect. A long tail will be present with normal viscosity and when expressed slightly faster, the fluid may well cling to the open end of the test tube as it receives the fluid (Fig. 3-1). Poor viscosity will be evident by a raindrop configuration with a short tail. Viscosity and hyaluronate

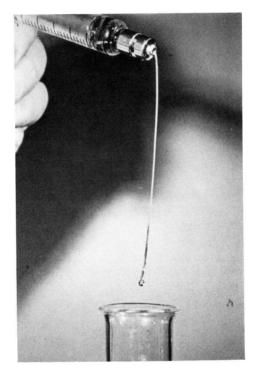

Fig. 3–1.   String test showing high (normal) viscosity.

concentration, which mirrors viscosity, can be measured in the laboratory by a variety of methods; however, they add little further information.[1-3]

Clinically, low viscosity is associated with inflammatory synovia, as in rheumatoid disease. This is caused by the depolymerization of the long chains of hyaluronate and can be further documented by the mucin clot test (to be discussed). Table 1-1 shows that viscosity is generally high in normal and noninflammatory synovia, for example, in osteoarthritis. There are numerous exceptions. Acute trauma with a sudden effusion or massive dependent edema about the involved joint will dilute the synovial hyaluronate and decrease viscosity in the absence of local inflammation. On the other hand, clotted white blood cells in an infected joint can lead to thickened joint fluid, although not truly a "normal" string test.

Combinations of disorders cause variations. What happens to a patient with hypothyroidism, where viscosity may be high, and concomitant inflammatory arthritis? What of a patient with inflammatory arthritis subsiding secondary to an intra-articular corticosteroid injection? Therefore, evaluation of viscosity adds some information, but other studies are more definitive.

COLOR (Plate 1)

Another bedside evaluation is color. Because most syringes are now translucent plastic, the tests for color and clarity should be performed in a clear glass tube. The green stoppered vacutainer commonly used in many hospitals and laboratories is normally coated with *sodium* heparin and is quite satisfactory. Do not use *lithium* heparin or oxalate as an anticoagulant, since these form crystals in joint fluid, causing confusion on microscopic examination. Samples of less than 1 ml may have their cellular detail disrupted by dilution with a liquid anticoagulant; in this case, it is preferable to carry the fluid in the syringe to the laboratory for prompt analysis.

Assuming a volume of greater than 1 ml, remove the test tube stopper and express the synovia into the tube, recap it, and gently tilt and roll the tube until the anticoagulant dissolves. Do not push the needle through the vacutainer stopper, as this adds unnecessary trauma to the cells and eliminates viscosity evaluation. Using a white background, judge the color. As noted in Table 1-1, normal fluid is colorless; noninflammatory and inflammatory fluids are yellowish or straw colored. The coloring is derived from the breakdown of red blood cells (RBCs) that have entered the joint cavity from the capillary bed just beneath the synovial lining cells. Irritation and inflammation of the synovium enhance diapedesis of RBCs. Subsequently, they break down, liberating heme, which degrades to bilirubin, producing xanthochromia. This occurs in Group I as well as Group II fluids and is analogous to the events that occur in spinal fluid after hemorrhage.

Septic fluid will have variable coloring depending on the infecting organism, the chromogens produced, and the intensity of the reaction, including the numbers of WBCs and RBCs present. Pus similar to that seen in an abscess is present if the infection is severe. A high concentration of rice bodies, products of degenerating proliferative synovial lining cells, or large numbers of crystals can mimic pus on gross examination.

Hemorrhagic fluid has a homogeneous distribution of blood that has not clotted, as compared with a traumatic puncture, in which the blood will lack homogeneity in the aspirated synovia, and, if in any great amount, it will clot. If pure blood appears in the syringe, usually the best approach is to withdraw the needle promptly, apply local pressure, and immediately seek another approach to the joint using a new sterile needle and syringe to aspirate the joint fluid. Usually, the fluid will not be hemorrhagic in a homogeneous fashion, thus securing evidence that the initial tap was traumatic. If, however, this second arthrocentesis produces the same bloody fluid as the first, that is good evidence in favor of a hemorrhagic fluid. To confirm this, an hematocrit can be performed on the synovia, comparing it with the peripheral blood hematocrit. The hematocrit will be the same in both samples if a vein rather than the joint cavity was entered; otherwise, the joint fluid hematocrit will be lower.

The clinical significance of a hemorrhagic fluid warrants a careful differentiation between a traumatic tap and grossly bloody synovia (Plate 1).

CLARITY

Clarity of synovia relates to the number and type of particles within it. Generally, WBCs are the most common particles present that change normally transparent fluid to translucent or opaque

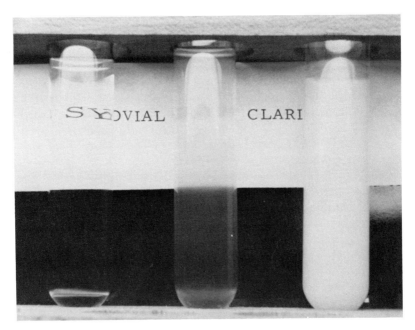

Fig. 3–2. Clarity test shows (left to right) transparent, translucent, and opaque fluids.

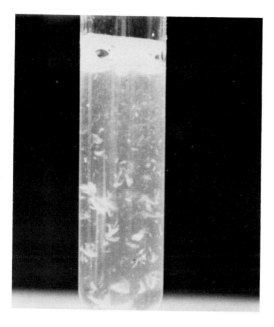

Fig. 3–3.   Rice bodies in test tube of joint fluid.

fluid (Table 1-1). Massive numbers of crystals, such as urate, calcium pyrophosphate, or cholesterol, occasionally occur in the absence of white cells, producing an opaque opalescent fluid. There is a filmy, shimmering, "oily" quality to the cholesterol crystals. Large numbers of RBCs will produce a "smoky" appearance, as in hematuria.

To test for clarity, place black printed material with a white background behind the clear glass tube of synovia in the presence of good lighting. If the print can be read through the joint fluid, it is transparent; if the difference between the black print and the white paper can be discerned only as light and dark, then it is translucent; if nothing can be seen through the fluid, it is opaque (Fig. 3–2).

Rarer causes of altered color and clarity are seen. Heavy fibrin deposits and free-floating tissue aggregates (rice bodies) can simulate clumps of WBCs (Fig. 3–3). Metal and plastic fragments in joint effusions following joint prosthesis implantation produce dark particles that generally fall to the bottom of the test tube on standing.[4,5] "Ground pepper" debris can be seen in the synovia of patients with ochronosis (Fig. 3–4).[6]

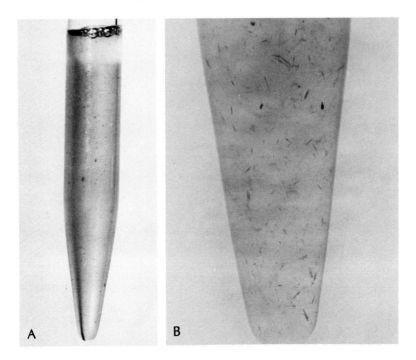

Fig. 3-4. "Ground pepper" sign in ochronosis. *A,* Joint fluid in test tube. *B,* Higher magnification of ochronotic shards. (Courtesy of Dungan A. Gordon, M.D., Toronto, Canada.)

REFERENCES

1. Ropes, M.W., and Bauer, W.: *Synovial Fluid Changes in Joint Disease.* Cambridge, Massachusetts, Harvard University Press, 1953.
2. Hasselbacher, P.: Measuring synovial fluid viscosity with a white blood cell diluting pipette. Arthritis Rheum., *19*:1358, 1978.
3. Bitter, T., and Muir, H.M.: A modified uranic acid carbazole reaction. Anal. Biochem., *4*:330, 1962.
4. Kitridou, R., Schumacher, H.R., Sbarbaro, J.L., and Hollander, J.L.: Recurrent hemarthrosis after prosthetic knee arthroplasty: Identification of metal particles in the synovial fluid. Arthritis Rheum., *12*:520, 1969.
5. Tong, I., Kaufman, R., and Beardmore, T.: Prosthetic synovitis. Presented, American Rheumatism Association Regional Meeting, Salt Lake City, 1980.
6. Hunter, T., Gordon, D.A., and Ogryzlo, M.A.: The ground pepper sign of synovial fluid; a new diagnostic feature of ochronosis. J. Rheum., *1*:45, 1974.

Chapter 4

The Total and Differential White Blood Cell Count

TOTAL WHITE BLOOD CELL COUNT

Tables 1–1 and 4–1 indicate the ranges and mean value for WBC and differential counts seen in normal and abnormal synovia. Although there is considerable overlap, these values are more reliable than the other differentiating criteria discussed thus far and are useful for serial evaluations in septic arthritis under treatment.

The techniques are identical to peripheral blood counts, except that automated counters may give false results by counting extracellular material and fat or become clogged by fluids more viscous than blood.[1] Newer counters use solutions that seem to give accurate results and are recommended for synovia, such as Haema-lyse 100 and Haema-line. At this time, however, caution is rec-

Table 4–1. *Mean Normal Joint Fluid WBC and Differential Values*[5]

	Mean Joint Fluid Values
WBC/mm³	63
Differential WBC (%)	
PMN	7
Lymphocytes	24
Monocytes	48
Macrophages	10
Synovial lining cells	4

ommended. Dual samples should be run using manual counts to check against your own automated counter until the WBC count is reproducible. WBC counts below 1000 mm^3 may be inaccurate. Also, acetic acid cannot be used as the diluent for manual counting as it will clot synovial protein by denaturation. WBCs become trapped in the clot, producing a falsely low WBC count. Therefore, it is still more reliable to count WBCs by hand using normal saline solution (0.85%) in the standard WBC pipette. If there are enough RBCs to make counting difficult, then lyse them using 0.3 N hypotonic saline as the diluent instead of normal saline. A small amount of 0.1% methylene blue can be added to the saline used as diluent to facilitate differentiation of WBCs from other cells and particles. The methylene blue alternatively can be added to the counting chamber.

It is important to record the presence of clots so that the clinician knows that the recorded WBC count is falsely low. The form devised for recording laboratory data is presented (Fig. 4-1).

DIFFERENTIAL WBC COUNT

The differential WBC count is performed in a standard fashion. Wright's stain requires no special adaptation. To maintain cell integrity, however, the smear should be made as soon as the joint fluid is received, even at night in the hospital laboratory. Staining of the air-dried smear then can be delayed, if necessary, without excessive loss of cell morphology. The smear should be made as thin as possible. The viscosity of the joint fluid tends to create thick smears containing smudged cells and excessive extracellular stain, which are difficult to interpret. If the total WBC count is low, spin down the specimen tube to sediment the cellular portion; usually 7 to 10 minutes at 3000 rpm is sufficient. Remove the supernatant and reconstitute the sediment with a few drops of supernatant. Make the smear from this preparation.

The smear for differential count will show cells seen in peripheral blood smears, PMNs, small lymphocytes, monocytes, eosinophils, and normal or abnormal RBCs. In addition, there may be synovial lining cells, macrophages, Reiter's cells, LE cells, large (stimulated) mononuclear cells, plasma cells, bone marrow spicules, bacterial inclusions, cytoplasmic inclusion vacuoles (see Chapter 7), and crystal outlines within phagocytic cells (Plate 2 and Figures 4–2 and 4–3).[2,3] WBC and PMN levels normally are low, but increase with inflammation and infection. Much information is gained from

SYNOVIANALYSIS
Report Form

Name _____ Date _____
Joint Aspirated _____ Time _____AM
PM

Group I ____ ; Group II ____ ; Group III ____ ; Hemorrhagic ____
Volume (ml): _____
Viscosity: High _____ ; Low _____
Color: Clear _____ ; Xanthrochromic _____ ; Opalescent _____ ;
    Other _____
Clarity: Transparent _____ ; Translucent _____ ; Opaque _____
Crystals: None _____ ; Few _____ ; Moderate _____ ; Many _____
    Elongation: Positive _____ ; Negative _____ ; Indeterminate _____
    Brightness: Weak _____ ; Strong _____
    Morphology: Rod ____ %; Rhomboid ____ %; Other ____ %
    Intracellular: _____ %; Extracellular: _____ %
    Extinction: On axis _____ ; Gradual _____
    Crystal Identity: MSUM ____ ; CPPD ____ ; Corticosteroid ____ ;
        Other _____
    Cytoplasmic Inclusion Bodies: _____
    Fibrils: _____
Total WBC/mm^3: _____
    PMN _____ %
    Lymphocytes
        Small _____ %
        Large _____ %
    Monocytes _____ %
    Macrophages _____ %
    Synovial lining cells _____ %
    Other _____ %
RBCs: Few _____ ; Many _____ ; TNTC _____
    Morphology: Normal _____ ; Other _____

Examined by: _____ Date: _____ Time: _____AM
PM

Fig. 4–1. Synovianalysis Report form.

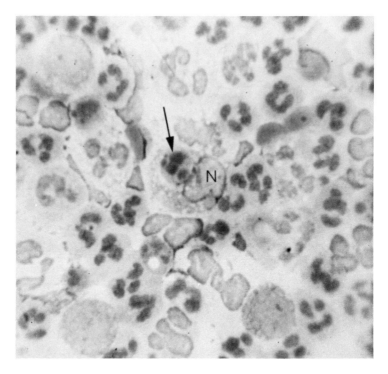

Fig. 4–2. "Reiter's cell." Photomicrograph of phagocytic mononuclear cell with nucleus *(N)* that has phagocytized a polymorphonuclear leukocyte (arrow). (From Schumacher, H.R.: Synovial fluid analysis. In *Textbook of Rheumatology.* Edited by William Kelley. Philadelphia, W.B. Saunders Co., 1981.

noting the presence, absence, and percentages of these cells (see Tables 1–1 and 1–2).

RBC morphology can be important when abnormal forms are seen, e.g., sickle cells.

Fluid from bursal and tendon sheaths is handled in the same fashion, although bursal fluid generally is not as reactive as joint fluid when responding to the same stimulus.[4] Remember, after such careful observation, to accurately record the data obtained.

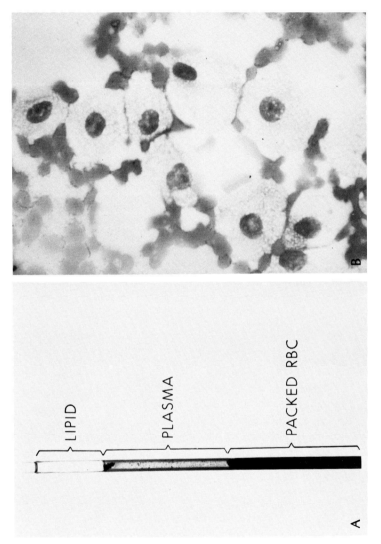

Fig. 4–3. Bone marrow spicules in joint fluid after fracture. *A,* Supernatant lipid layer in micro-hematocrit tube after centrifugation of bloody joint fluid (gross). *B,* Marrow fat cells in joint fluid. Wright's stain; original magnification ×1000, ×3.6. (From Lawrence, C., and Seife, B.: Bone marrow in joint fluid. Ann. Intern. Med., 74:740, 1971.)

REFERENCES

1. Vincent, J., Korn, J.H., Podewell, C., and Tully, E.: Synovial fluid pseudoleukocytosis. Arthritis Rheum., *12*:1399, 1980.
2. Lawrence, C., and Seifo,B.: Bone marrow in joint fluid: A clue to fracture. Ann. Intern. Med., *74*:740, 1971.
3. Good, A.E., and Fishette, W.A.: Crystals in dried smears of synovial fluid. JAMA, *198*:198, 1966.
4. Canoso, J.J., and Yood, R.A.: Reaction of superficial bursae in response to specific disease stimuli. Arthritis Rheum., *12*:1361, 1979.
5. Adapted from McCarty, D.J.: *Arthritis and Allied Conditions.* 9th Edition. Philadelphia, Lea & Febiger, 1979.

Chapter 5

Wet Preparation

A "wet preparation" is a microscopic slide prepared for the purpose of examining whole joint fluid under the microscope.

Essential materials are a clean slide, a clean cover slip, clear nail polish, and a clean Pasteur pipette or bacteriologic loop. The sooner the fluid can be analyzed, the better. Cellular detail can be lost after as little as 2 hours.

Usually the joint fluid will come to the laboratory in a stoppered test tube. One commonly used tube is the green stoppered vacutainer, which has sodium heparin as the anticoagulant. Using non-anticoagulated tubes will cause the joint fluid to clot, thus trapping white cells and decreasing the white cell count. Lithium heparin and calcium oxalate, although anticoagulants, are not suitable as they form crystals that not only are then found free in the joint fluid, but that also may be phagocytosed by cells as well.[1,2] Therefore, as mentioned in a previous chapter, to avoid this confusion, use only *sodium* heparin or ethylenediaminetetraacetate (EDTA), which will not produce crystalline artifacts.

TECHNIQUE OF SLIDE PREPARATION

The glass slide and cover slip must be cleaned carefully; even dust and bits of lens paper have light-splitting (refractile) properties. Acetone cleansing and air drying are usually sufficient. Practically speaking, it is better to obtain precleaned slides and cover slips; however, even these must be carefully examined before use. The containing boxes must be kept covered once the box has been opened to keep dust out. Place the slide on a clean surface and lean the cover slip against it for ease of retrieval. Remove one drop of joint fluid from the tube with a flamed bacteriologic loop or a clean Pasteur pipette. If particles or clots are present, try to stir the fluid sufficiently to obtain a clot or a representative sample. Place the drop of fluid on the slide, cover with the cover slip, and seal with clear nail polish. The nail polish should be on the top surface of the *slide* and the *edge* of the cover slip and not on the top surface of the *cover slip*. This approach will prevent nail polish from touching the oil immersion objective lens when changing objectives. For this same reason, allow time for the polish to dry before viewing under the microscope. Sealing the cover slip to the slide on all four sides will decrease the streaming of cells and extracellular material, thus allowing more accurate observations. This will also retard dehydration of the joint fluid on the slide. The dehydration process can cause cellular disruption and de novo precipitation of MSUM crystals in fluid having a high urate concentration. These crystals even may be phagocytosed by viable cells, giving the false diagnosis of acute gout.

At times, joint fluid aspirated may be insufficient to draw up from the needle into the syringe. In this case, a "needle flush" should be performed. Detach the syringe from the needle, draw 2 to 3 ml of air into the syringe, reattach the needle, then force the air through the needle by pressing on the plunger briskly. With the needle bevel down over the center of the slide, minute droplets of fluid retained in the needle should be forced out onto the slide. Soft tissue aspirates may be handled in this same fashion.

Because the transparent droplets are so fine, it is sometimes difficult to find them under the microscope. It is useful, at times, to place a dot on the underside of the slide with a felt-tip pen near the droplet to help locate it.

If an air needle flush is not effective, a drop of alcohol may be passed through the needle. Although the water in the alcohol could dissolve urate crystals, it is our impression that crystals, when viewed immediately, remain intact.

If the total fluid volume is used for making a single wet preparation, after viewing under the polarized light microscope, the same slide can be used for a differential WBC count, either by phase light microscopy on the unstained specimen (Fig. 5–1),[3] or by removing the cover slip and performing a Wright's stain.

TISSUE SPECIMEN

The preparation of a tissue specimen, such as a renal biopsy suspected of containing urate tophi, for polarized light examination

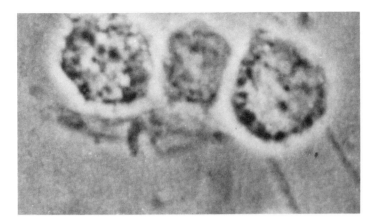

Fig. 5–1. Differential white blood count, unstained. Nuclei appear lighter; cytoplasm is darker. Phase light (× 1250). Left to right: Polymorphonuclear leukocyte, medium-sized lymphocyte, large mononuclear cell. (From Gatter, R.A., and Richmond, J.D.: Predominance of synovial fluid lymphocytes in early rheumatoid arthritis. J. Rheumatol., 2:340, 1975.)

is best performed on a fresh specimen not placed in any aqueous preservative. The fresh specimen should be transferred immediately for cryostat sectioning. Once frozen, the thinnest possible sections are placed directly on a clean slide. Usually, it is difficult to apply a cover slip over the section. Rather, use low power, medium, and high dry, if possible, to identify the sheaves of MSUM crystals (Plate 3).

REFERENCES

1. Gatter, R.A., and McCarty, D.J.: Synovianalysis. Rheumatism, *20*:2, 1964.
2. Tanphaichitr, K., Spilberg, I., and Hahn, B.: Letter to the editor. Lithium heparin crystals simulating calcium pyrophosphate dihydrate crystals in synovial fluid. Arthritis Rheum., *19*:966-968, 1976.
3. Jones, R.M.: *McClung's Handbook of Microscopical Technique.* 3rd Edition. New York, Paul Hoeber, Inc., 1950, pp. 571–585.

Chapter 6

Clinical Application of the Compensated Polarized Light and Phase Light Microscope

Microscopic synovianalysis requires a compensated polarized light microscope with $10 \times$, $40 \times$, and $100 \times$ (oil immersion) objectives. A phase condenser and an oil immersion phase objective are highly recommended.

The purpose of microscopic examination is to detect pathologic material in joint fluid. In particular, the finding of calcium pyrophosphate dihydrate (CPPD) and/or monosodium urate monohydrate (MSUM) crystals naturally occurring in synovial fluid gives the instant diagnosis of pseudogout or gout, respectively. This is one of the few pathognomonic tests in the study of the rheumatic diseases. Therefore, when present, these crystals must be recognized and reported.

In Chapter 12, the detailed optics are discussed, but at this point a few practical notes are needed to understand what will be observed (Fig. 6–1).

The purpose of the lower polarizing plate (the polarizer) is to orient the microscope's light into many parallel planes (plane-polarized light). If a second similar plate (the analyzer) is turned 90° to these parallel light planes, *no* light will pass through the second plate. Therefore, the eye sees a dark microscopic field (Fig.

31

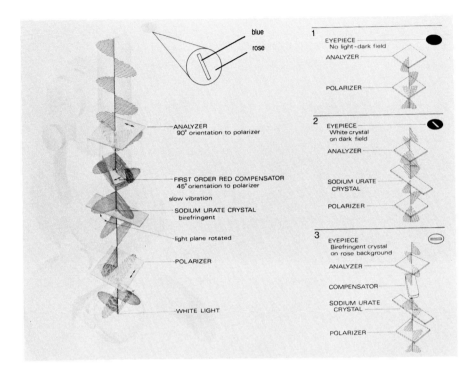

Fig. 6–1. Light path of compensated polarizing microscope. Composite (left) and components (right). (From Gatter, R.A.: The compensated polarized light microscope in clinical rheumatology. Arthritis Rheum., *17*:253, 1974.)

6–1–1). If a wet preparation containing crystals is placed between these polarizing plates, the direction of the light planes will be altered sufficiently by passing through these crystals to allow the light to slip through the analyzer. Now the eye sees white light in the shape of the crystals on a dark field (Fig. 6-1-2). By also placing a first-order red compensator in the light path between the polarizer and the analyzer, the field becomes rose colored, and the crystals turn blue or yellow depending on their identity and their orientation to the compensator's direction of slow vibration (Fig. 6–1–3). This direction is indicated by a line marked on the compensator, usually with the Greek letter, γ (gamma) (Fig. 6–1, left column).

Crystals are most commonly needle shaped (rod) (acicular). Turn a rotating microscope stage until the crystal's physical long axis is parallel to the orienting line of the compensator, and note the color. This process is called *elongation*. If, in this position, the crystal is *blue,* it has a positive optic sign, or *positive elongation,* for example, CPPD. If, in this position, the crystal is *yellow,* it exhibits a negative optic sign, or *negative elongation,* for example, MSUM. These two common pathologic crystals demonstrate the basics necessary for crystal differentiation under this microscope. A mnemonic is useful to recall this information. YUN-BPP (pronounced "Yun-bip") stands for Yellow-Urate-Negative; Blue-Pyrophosphate-Positive.[1] This applies when the crystal's long axis is parallel to the compensator's orienting line.

Throughout the rheumatology literature, positive and negative "birefringence" are terms commonly used to mean positive and negative elongation. Birefringence cannot be positive or negative. What is meant, but not said, is that the crystal is *birefringent,* that is, having two optical axes, and that the *optic sign* is *positive* or *negative.* The optic sign is the important differentiating feature, and elongation is the process used to determine it. Therefore, positive or negative elongation is the preferred term.

In the composite microscopic light path depicting compensated polarized light using the example of a MSUM crystal (left side of Figure 6–1), note that the crystal is *blue* when *perpendicular* to the slow vibration orientation of the compensator. When turned 90°, it will be *yellow* and *parallel.* In both cases, negative elongation is indicated.

Rotating either MSUM or CPPD crystals 90° will cause them to change from yellow to blue or from blue to yellow. There are only two colors to deal with. Midway between, on the axes of the polarizer and the analyzer, there will be a zone in which no blue or yellow color will be seen at all, called *extinction.* MSUM has crisp extinction; CPPD has a slower transition or "oblique extinction," as discussed in another chapter (Fig. 6–2).

A phase objective and phase condenser are recommended as valuable adjuncts for synovianalysis. Phase light is diffused light, not oriented directly on the line of sight, and thereby it produces highlights and shadows on margins of cellular structures that are difficult to see by white or polarized light. Thus, it is most helpful when observing cells and their contents, such as cytoplasmic inclusion bodies, cell nuclei, and small intracellular crystals, that cannot be seen otherwise.

VIEWING TECHNIQUES

Long periods of scanning cause fatigue, frustration, and, ultimately, less accurate observations; this is generally not necessary.

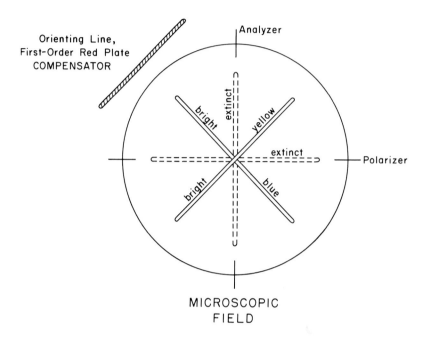

Fig. 6–2. Microscopic field with monosodium urate monohydrate crystal rotating 360° under compensated polarized light. Maximum brilliance occurs parallel and perpendicular to the compensator; extinction occurs in the plane of the polarizer and analyzer.

Assuming that the microscope is fully equipped with polarizer, analyzer, first-order red compensator, ordinary light and phase objectives, phase contrast condenser, and rotating stage, our experience has been that the most effective initial approach to a slide is scanning under low power (10× objective) with compensated polarized light. Vary the light intensity via light source and condenser iris for best vision, but not too bright, thus "washing out" the crystals. With the naked eye, look for the test material or a bubble; place this area on the stage in the center of the light path. If a small amount is present, this is difficult to do; the ink dot marked on the underside of the slide, noted before, will help. Focus on the test material. If focusing to the correct depth is still difficult, move the slide so that the edge of the cover slip is in view, and focus on it. Frequently, trapped air bubbles, streaming of cells, increased cell concentration, or precipitated nail polish that is refractile along this edge will be of assistance.

Once focused on the slide's upper surface (not the artifacts on top of the cover slip or the bottom of the slide), scan under low power at random, looking for a cluster of cells and fibrils. Scrutinize such clumping for birefringent material in or about the cells by rotating the microscope stage 90° back and forth while fine focusing slightly up and down. To keep perspective, think that crystal length may be one tenth the diameter of a WBC. Thinking small will cause you to see more crystals promptly. Crystals will appear regularly shaped and will change colors from yellow to blue against the rose background. This flashing of light will draw attention to areas of the slide for higher-power examination.

Although high dry magnification (40×) many times may confirm crystal identification, a complete examination should include evaluation under oil immersion (100× objective). With a 10× to 12.5× eyepiece or a total of 1000× to 1250×, two-point discrimination should be 0.5 to 1.0 μm. This level of magnification is optimal. Many times a fluid that initially appears to have only a few crystals or none at all is found to have a large population of small crystals. At times, a second different crystal population is identified. Occasionally, it requires thorough searching of many cellular clumps with variation of light and condenser settings to find thin, flat crystals, particularly intracellular CPPD, which normally have less brilliance than MSUM. A phase oil immersion objective (100×) is helpful in this situation. Once one crystal is identified, seek out others to confirm your findings, then estimate the number of crystals of each type that are present as "few," "moderate," or "many," and estimate what percentage are intracellular and extracellular. A systematic screen is necessary for this, using standard patterns of your choice, until satisfied that a fair estimate is possible, taking the clumps of cells into account. These are helpful data for the clinician relating to acuteness of the arthritic process. Occasionally, a joint fluid will have so few cells and such sparse extracellular material that centrifugation of the fluid and microscopic examination of the button is necessary. This is a useful method; however, care must be taken to clearly record that the results were obtained from a concentrated specimen to avoid confusion.

REFERENCES

1. Phelps, P.: Personal communication.

Chapter 7

Microscopic Findings Under Compensated Polarized Light and Phase Light

REFRACTILE PATHOLOGIC FINDINGS

In the clinical setting, the important question is, "What is the unknown crystal: urate, calcium pyrophosphate, or some other refractile (light-bending) material?" For this answer, all available criteria are needed (Table 7–1).

Monosodium Urate Monohydrate (MSUM)

Most importantly, this crystal exhibits negative elongation. Its intensity (brightness) is strong. Its configuration is usually acicular (rod or needle shaped). Extinction (that point of rotation at which the crystal takes on the same color as the background, i.e., isotropic) occurs instantly and exactly on the axis of the polarizer and the analyzer (Fig. 6–2; Plate 4a, b, and c). In addition, "beachball" spherules of urate have been reported in synovia from gouty joints (Plate 5). These spherulites are actually made up of numerous acicular crystals radiating out from the center and therefore show some parallel and some perpendicular to the compensator's γ line at all times.[1]

Table 7–1. *Joint Fluid Crystal Characteristics*

Crystal	Elongation	Brightness (Intensity)	Morphology	Extinction	Size (Estimates)
MSUM	Negative	Strong	Rod, spherule	On axis sharply	Submicroscopic-40 μm
CPPD	Positive	Weak	Rod and rhomboid	Gradual	Submicroscopic-40 μm
HA			Hexagonal individual crystals "Cluster of shiny coins"		Submicroscopic (240 Å) to clusters 1.9–15.6 μm
CaHPO$_4$ 2H$_2$O	Positive	Strong	Rod		
Cholesterol	Negative Detection difficult	Weak	Plates (notched corners) Few rods		5–40 μm
Lipid inclusions	Maltese cross		Round intracellular inclusions		0.5–1 μm
Lipid liquid	Maltese cross		Round extracellular		
Calcium oxalate	Positive Detection difficult	Variable Weak	Tetrahedron Rods		
Lithium heparin	Positive	Weak	Polymorphic		2–5 μm
Talc	Maltese cross	Strong	Ovoid		
Corticosteroid	Variable	Usually strong	Polymorphic		1–40 μm
Nail polish	Positive	Strong	Rod		5–10 μm
Immersion oil	Positive	Strong	Polymorphic		1–5 μm

Calcium Pyrophosphate Dihydrate (CPPD)

Most importantly, this crystal exhibits positive elongation. Its intensity is weak, causing less brilliant color than is noted with MSUM crystals. Its configuration is either acicular or rhomboid (six surfaces, each a parallelogram, with opposite surfaces alike). The two morphologic forms frequently are present in nearly equal numbers, although one or the other may predominate. Great care must be taken to avoid missing crystals with intensity so weak that they are nearly isotropic; phase microscopy will help define these crystals. Extinction occurs gradually as the crystal passes the axes of the polarizer and the analyzer (Plate 6a and b). Frequently, smaller intracellular CPPD crystals will be seen within vacuoles. This is not true of MSUM crystals, which tend to disrupt the enclosing membrane secondary to adherence to the crystal surface.

The diagnoses of gout and pseudogout are made by identifying the MSUM and CPPD crystals, respectively.

Crystal size and morphology are not as important as optical sign and brightness; however, all available parameters should be used to ensure the most accurate report. This is particularly true because new observations of synovial contents continue to be made. There is no assurance that what is being observed will fit into a category already described. Keep alert to fine differences; you may make a new observation. Crystals can be any length, from submicroscopic to greater than five times the diameter of a PMN. Exceptions do occur. One sample of crystals removed surgically from a carpal tunnel was referred for evaluation because all the crystals were rhomboids with strong negative elongation. They proved to be MSUM on x-ray diffraction. This unusual morphology was thought to relate to the compressed soft tissue location and other local factors as compared with joint fluid.

Hydroxyapatite (HA)

Other pathologic crystals are found in man. Hydroxyapatite (HA) crystals from periarticular structures were seen, both extracellular and within PMNs, as "shiny coins" under phase contrast microscopy, measuring 3 to 65 μm in diameter (Fig. 7–1a).[2] Later, similar shiny inclusions under polarized light were found to stain purple on Wright's staining of synovial lining cells in joint fluid; this patient had acute arthritis associated with electron microscopic findings of HA crystals (Fig. 7–1b).[3] Alizarin Red S, which stains calcium compounds, adds further information (Plate 7).[4] Others confirmed HA-associated acute arthritis by submicroscopic meth-

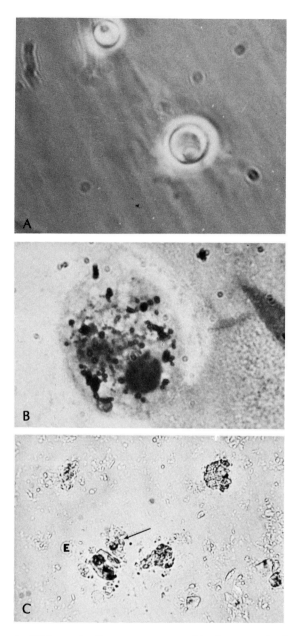

Fig. 7–1. *A,* "Shiny coins" are aggregates of hydroxyapatite in periarticular tissue. Size varies from 3 to 65 μm (phase light, ×1250). (From
McCarty, D.J., and Gatter, R.A.: Recurrent acute inflammation associated
with focal apatite crystal deposition. Arthritis Rheum., *9:*804, 1966.) *B,*
Joint fluid intracellular hydroxyapatite clumps which are purple on
Wright's stain. Ordinary light (×850). (From Schumacher, H.R.: Pathogenesis of crystal-induced synovitis. In *Crystal Induced Arthropathies.* Clinics
in Rheumatic Diseases. Edited by William Kelley. Vol. 3. London, W.B.
Saunders, 1977.) *C,* Shiny hydroxyapatite aggregate (arrow) within a joint
fluid leukocyte. Erythrocyte (E). Compensated polarized light (×1000).
(Courtesy of H. Ralph Schumacher, M.D.)

ods, but without findings on light microscopy.[5] Recently, a syndrome characterized by rotator cuff defects, arthritis, active collagenase, and neutral protease has been reported to contain joint fluid HA crystal spheroidal masses 1.9 to 15.6 μm in diameter, which seem to be the stimulating factor.[6] Elbow and finger erosive arthropathy has been described associated with HA crystals (Fig. 7–1c).[7] Therefore, large clumps of HA can be suspected by light microscopy, but electron microscopy and chemical testing are required for conclusive proof.

Calcium Hydrogen Phosphate Dihydrate

Calcium hydrogen phosphate dihydrate was initially found in menisci of cadavers.[8,9] Three other reports suggest that calcium hydrogen phosphate dihydrate is involved in synovitis and arthritis.[10–12] This crystal is bright and exhibits positive elongation (Plate 8).

Calcium Oxalate

Recently, calcium oxalate crystals have been found to form in chronic dialysis patients.[13]

Cholesterol Crystals

Cholesterol crystals, although not a stimulus to inflammation, do occur in joint and bursal fluids.[14] Morphologically, they are nearly equilateral plates that adhere to one another's surfaces. When viewed in these stacks, there is a characteristic appearance of notched corners (Plate 9). Some of this is real, but some is caused by the irregular stacking of regular crystals (Plate 10). Acicular (rod) morphology is less frequently seen. These single crystals are of weak intensity (brightness), although moderately bright when in stacks. They are extracellular and large, and negative elongation may be detected.

Lipid

Lipid inclusions within leukocytes have been reportedly associated with a case of inflammatory monoarthritis. The inclusions were visible only under polarized light.[15] Fracture through the joint must also be considered. Larger "lipid liquid" crystals also have been seen extracellularly associated with acute arthritis (Plate 11).[16]

Cryoprotein

Crystals of IgG lambda cryoprotein were recovered from joint fluid, synovial tissue, Bowman's membrane, and serum at 4° C in

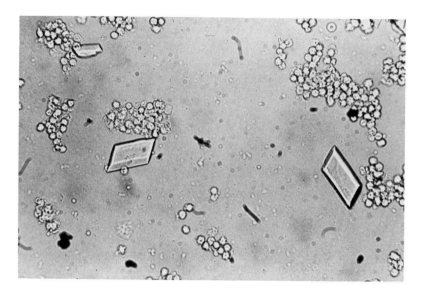

Fig. 7–2. Crystals of IgG Lambda cryoprotein from joint fluid of a patient with peripheral erosive arthritis and tenosynovitis. Crystals are 50 μm × 25 μm with positive and negative elongation. (Courtesy of R.L. Dawkins, M.D.)

a patient with peripheral erosive arthritis and tendonitis (Fig. 7–2).[17]

Amyloid

Amyloid fragments have been identified in joint fluid. Congo red positive areas show green birefringence under polarized light (Fig. 7–3).[18]

Thorns

Plant thorns have not been reported in joint fluid, but have been embedded in synovial membrane, causing synovitis. They are birefringent and have varying fragmented shapes.[19]

REFRACTILE ARTIFACTS

Artifacts are important findings in joint fluid and several are refractile. Familiarity with commonly seen pathologic crystals is most helpful. In most instances, the experienced observer will suspect artifact when the combination of size, morphology, brightness, and optic sign are not usual.

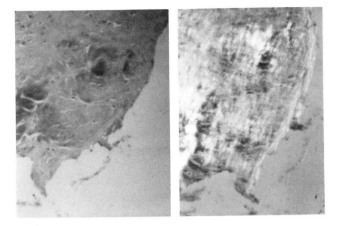

Fig. 7–3. Amyloid deposits in synovial lining fragments in joint fluid. Congo red positive stain under ordinary light (left) and showing refractile qualities under polarized light (right) ×600. (From Gordon, D.A., Pruzanski, W., and Ogryzlo, M.A.: Synovial fluid examination for the diagnosis of amyloidosis. Ann. Rheum. Dis., 32:428, 1973.)

Calcium Oxalate

Calcium oxalate crystals form in joint fluid that has been placed in a test tube containing oxalate as an anticoagulant. The crystals are usually cubic, and the optic sign is usually not ascertainable, although positive elongation would be expected; brightness is quite variable (Plate 12).[20,21]

Lithium Heparin

Lithium heparin (not sodium heparin), also an anticoagulant, will crystallize with positive elongation. The shape is variable, and they are usually small (2 to 5 μm) (Plate 13).[22,23]

Both calcium oxalate and lithium crystals may be phagocytosed by PMNs.

Talc

Occasionally, talc from surgical gloves will appear in joint fluid as bright maltese crosses (Plate 14).

Corticosteroid

The most common artifact, in our experience, has been slowly absorbed corticosteroid crystals, which may be present weeks, even months, after an intra-articular injection. Similarly, corticosteroid crystals can contaminate synovia by withdrawing joint fluid from the joint or discharging it into the test tube through a needle that has been used to draw up corticosteroid medication. Some of these crystals have distinguishing characteristics (Plate 15).

Prosthetic Fragments

Metal fragments from worn prostheses have been noted in synovia.[24] Although this metal component is not refractile, fractured polymethylmethacrylate and ultrahigh-molecular-weight polyethylene debris in synovial membrane biopsies from joints containing prostheses are birefringent.[25] Recently, polyethylene fragments were reported in synovia as well (Fig. 7–4).[26]

Nail Polish

Nail polish used to seal the cover slip for a wet preparation can deposit large numbers of bright rods with positive elongation at the margin of the cover slip.

Immersion Oil

Immersion oil may contain crystals with a wide variety of shapes and sizes, frequently in the smaller range, showing positive elongation. Of course, if properly focused under the cover slip, not on top of it, these crystals will not be seen or be a source of confusion.

Dust and Fibers

Dust and fiber from lens paper are birefringent and are not regularly shaped. They are usually larger branching structures as compared with pathologic crystals.

NONREFRACTILE FINDINGS

These entities are best seen under phase light or, second best, by ordinary light with the condenser lowered. Noncrystalline natural material is found in synovia; although not generally stimuli for arthritis, they must be recognized.

Cartilage

Cartilage fragments are morphologically irregular and are not generally refractile, even though collagen fibrils within them are. This may relate to orderliness and/or to the mass of the fragment. Variable results can be expected (Fig. 7–5). The irregular shape will distinguish cartilage from crystals.

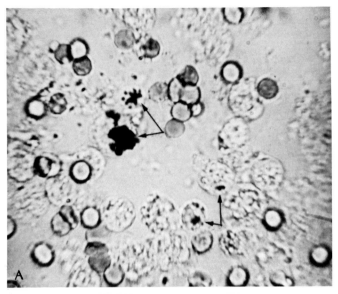

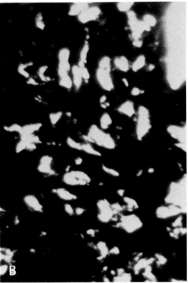

Fig. 7–4. *A,* Intracellular metal fragments (×750). (From Kitridou, R.C., Schumacher, H.R., Sbarbaro, J.L., and Hollander, J.L.: Recurrent hemarthrosis after prosthetic knee arthroplasty: identification of metal particles in synovial fluid. Arthritis Rheum., *12*:520, 1969.) *B,* Photomicrography of synovial membrane containing birefringent methylmethacrylate and polyethylene. Plane polarized light (×160). (From Crugnola, A., Schiller, A., and Radin, E.: Polymeric debris in synovium after total hip replacement: histological identification. J. Bone Joint Surg., *59A*:860, 1977.)

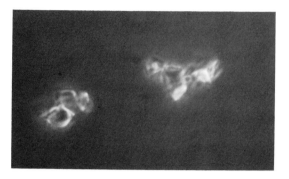

Fig. 7–5. Cartilage fragments. Compensated polarized light (×1250).

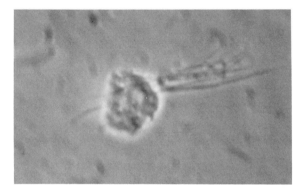

Fig. 7–6. Fibrils with overlying white blood cell. Phase light (×1250).

Fibrin and Fibrils

Fibrin will appear in wisps that are nonbirefringent, but that can, when rather straight, appear morphologically like a fine, needle-shaped crystal. Careful observation, however, will show them to be irregular, branching, or curved. Some of these strands are collagen fibrils also, but can be differentiated only by electron microscopy (Fig. 7–6).[27]

Silastic Fragments

Silastic fragments from joint replacements, usually for small joints of hands and feet, are not birefringent.[26]

Ochronosis

In ochronosis, synovia may contain gold-colored cartilaginous shards (shown grossly in Chapter 3).[28]

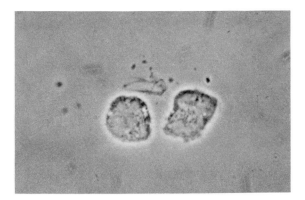

Fig. 7–7. Cytoplasmic inclusion bodies (CIB). Note the peripheral location of the vacuoles and the eccentric dark granules. Phase light (× 1250).

PHASE CONTRAST

Changing to the phase contrast condenser and to phase objective while still viewing under compensated polarizing light allows a view of crystals within cells with some coloring. This is helpful for defining questionable intracellular crystals. Removing the polarizer or analyzer from the light path, however, gives better definition. All the unstained cells and extracellular material, mentioned under the section on Wright's stain, are better seen under phase contrast.

Cytoplasmic Inclusion Bodies (CIB) and Crystals

CIB stand out, as do fibrils, fibrin, and cartilage (Fig. 7–7). As mentioned earlier, a differential WBC can be done by noting nuclear patterns. Morphology of RBCs also is easier to define.

Phase contrast offers the ability to observe the dynamics of phagocytosis and cell motility as the pseudopods of living cells are evident and mobile. This is equally true for intracellular contents of the cytoplasm. A new appreciation for the number of small and less brilliant crystals present in one cell will develop.

REFERENCES

1. Fiechtner, J.J., and Simkin, P.A.: Urate spherulites in gouty synovia. JAMA, 245:1533, 1981.
2. McCarty, D.J., and Gatter, R.A.: Recurrent acute inflammation associated with focal apatite crystal deposition. Arthritis Rheum., 9:804, 1966.
3. Schumacher, H.R., Somlyo, A.P., Tse, R.L., and Maurer, K.: Apatite crystal associated with arthritis. Ann. Intern. Med., 87:411, 1977.

4. Paul, H., Reginato, A.J., Schumacher, H.R.: Alizarin red S staining as a screening test to detect calcium compounds in synovial fluid. Arthritis Rheum., 26:191, 1983.
5. Dieppe, P.A., Crocker, P., Huskisson, E.C., and Willoughby, D.A.: Apatite deposition disease. Lancet, 1:266, 1976.
6. McCarty, D.J., et al.: Milwaukee shoulder: Association of microspheroids containing hydroxyapatite crystals, active collagenase, and neutral protease with rotator cuff defects. I. Clinical aspects. Arthritis Rheum., 24:464, 1981.
7. Schumacher, H.R., Miller, J.L., Ludivico, C., and Jessar, R.A.: Erosive arthritis associated with apatite crystal deposition. Arthritis Rheum., 24:31, 1981.
8. McCarty, D.J., and Gatter, R.A.: Identification of calcium hydrogen phosphate dihydrate crystals in human fibrocartilage. Nature, 201:391, 1963.
9. McCarty, D.J., Hogan, J.M., Gatter, R.A., and Grossman, M.: Studies on pathological calcifications in human cartilage. J. Bone Joint Surg., 48:303, 1966.
10. Skinner, M., and Cohen, A.S.: Calcium pyrophosphate dihydrate crystal deposition disease. Arch. Intern. Med., 123:636, 1969.
11. Gaucher, A., et al.: Identification des cristaux observés dans les arthropathies destructrices de la chondrocalcinose. Rev. Rhum., 44:407, 1977.
12. Utsinger, P.D.: Dicalcium phosphate deposition disease; a suspected new crystal-induced arthritis. Presented 14th International Congress of Rheumatology, San Francisco, June, 1977.
13. Hoffman, G.S., et al.: Calcium oxalate microcrystalline arthritis in end stage renal disease. Arthritis Rheum., 24:73, 1981 (Abstract).
14. Zuckner, J., Uddin, J., Gantner, G.E., and Dorner, R.W.: Cholesterol crystals in synovial fluid. Ann. Intern. Med., 60:436, 1964.
15. Weinstein, J.: Synovial fluid leukocytosis associated with intracellular lipid inclusions. Arch. Intern. Med., 140:560, 1980.
16. Reginato, H.J., Schumacher, H.R., Allan, D., and Rabinowitz, J.L.: Acute monoarthritis associated with lipid liquid crystals. Arthritis Rheum., 25:535, 1982 (Abstract).
17. Langlands, D.R., et al.: Arthritis associated with a crystallizing cryoprecipitable IgG paraprotein. Am. J. Med., 68:461, 1980.
18. Gordon, D.A., Pruzanski, W., and Ogryzlo, M.A.: Synovial fluid examination for the diagnosis of amyloidosis. Ann. Rheum. Dis., 32:428, 1973.
19. Sugarman, M., Stobie, D.G., Quismorio, F.P., and Hanson, V.: Plant thorn synovitis. Presented, 40th Annual Meeting, American Rheumatism Association, Chicago, 1976.
20. Gatter, R.A., and McCarty, D.J.: Synovianalysis, a rapid clinical diagnostic procedure. Rheumatism, 20:2, 1964.
21. Gatter, R.A.: Use of the compensated polarizing microscope. In *Crystal Induced Arthropathies.* Clinics in Rheumatic Diseases. Edited by William Kelley. Vol. 3. London, W.B. Saunders, 1977.
22. Tanphaichitr, K., Spilberg, I., and Hahn, B.: Lithium heparin crystals simulating calcium pyrophosphate dihydrate crystals in synovial fluid. Arthritis Rheum., 19:966, 1976 (Letter).

23. Schumacher, H.R.: Synovial fluid analysis. In *Textbook of Rheumatology.* Edited by William Kelley, et al. Philadelphia, W.B. Saunders, 1981.
24. Kitridou, R.C., Schumacher, H.R., Sbarbaro, J.L., and Hollander, J.L.: Recurrent hemarthrosis after prosthetic knee arthroplasty: Identification of metal particles in the synovial fluid. Arthritis Rheum., *12*:520, 1969.
25. Crugnola, A., Schiller, A., and Radin, E.: Polymeric debris in synovium after total hip replacement: histological identification. J. Bone Joint Surg., *59A*:860, 1977.
26. Tong, I., Kaufman, R., and Beardmore, T.: Prosthetic synovitis. Presented, American Rheumatism Association Regional Meeting, Salt Lake City, 1980.
27. Kitridou, R.C., et al.: Identification of collagen in synovial fluid. Arthritis Rheum., *12*:580, 1969.
28. Schumacher, H.R., and Holdsworth, D.E.: Ochronotic arthropathy. I. Clinicopathologic studies. Semin. Arthritis Rheum., *6*:207, 1977.

Chapter 8

Stains, Cultures, and Other Tests For Infection

STAINS

Staining of synovia is important for routine differential WBC counts. In addition, there are special stains that help define certain cell types. Table 8–1 indicates some of the more common stains used. As you will note, usually no special handling is required, and the staining procedure is not altered specifically for joint fluid. The authors who have contributed to our knowledge of staining are too numerous to report; only a few are mentioned.[1-3]

The Gram stain cannot be overemphasized (Plate 16). When sepsis is at all possible, a Gram stain and routine aerobic and anaerobic culture should always be obtained. If tuberculosis is suspected, then a Ziehl-Neelsen stain should be performed along with culture. If cells are sparse, centrifugation, as discussed earlier, will be helpful. Stains for organisms, if positive, can alert the physician to institute antibiotic therapy before cultures have produced growth and thereby decrease the potential for irreversible joint damage.

CULTURES

Routine, fungus, and tuberculosis cultures can be placed in a sterile culture tube for prompt transport to the laboratory for incubation on blood agar (or trypticase soy broth), Sabouraud's dextrose agar, and Löwenstein-Jensen medium, respectively (Table

Table 8–1. *Joint Fluid Stains**†

STAIN	SPECIAL TECHNIQUES	FINDINGS	APPEARANCE
Wright's	None	Diff. WBC Crystals	See Chapter 4. HA = purple CPPD = clear MSUM = background color
		Intracellular debris Intracellular ochronotic material Cryoproteins	Purple Brown Blue
Gram	None	Intracellular bacteria	Gram ± cocci or rods
Ziehl-Neelsen	None	Intracellular acid-fast bacilli	+ stained rods
Hematoxylin-eosin	Centrifuge, examine button	Tumor cells Rice bodies	Standard histology
Congo Red	Compensated polarized light examination	Amyloid deposits	Positive stain Birefringent tissue (green)
Oil Red O	None	Marrow, fat particles from joint fracture or pancreatitis	Positive stain
Prussian Blue	None	Intracellular iron (hemochromatosis, pigmented villonodular synovitis)	Positive stain
Alizarin red S	None	Calcium (HA clumps)	Positive stain
Von Kossa	None	CPPD, HA crystals (phosphate-bound calcium compounds)	Purple to brown
Alcian Blue	None	Intracellular mucopolysaccharides	Positive stain
Sudan Black	None	Large monocytes	Positive stain Nuclear:cytoplasmic ratio > 1
		Large lymphocytes (immunoblasts)	Negative stain Nuclear:cytoplasmic ratio > 1
		Synovial lining cells	Large cells, negative stain Nuclear:cytoplasmic ratio < 1, nucleus eccentric

*CPPD—calcium pyrophosphate dihydrate
MSUM—monosodium urate monohydrate
HA—hydroxyapatite
†Photographs of cells are in the section of color plates.

Table 8–2. *Joint Fluid Cultures*

ORGANISMS	MEDIA	SPECIAL PROCEDURES
Routine	Sheep blood agar Trypticase soy broth	None
Neisseria gonorrhoeae	Thayer-Martin Chocolate agar	Aerobic and anaerobic 2–10 days at 37° C (see text)
Anaerobes	Trypticase soy broth	Anaerobic (see text)
Fungi	Sabouraud's dextrose agar	None
Mycobacterium tuberculosis	Löwenstein-Jensen	Incubation for 6 weeks
Viruses	Animal inoculation	Contact your local viral reference laboratory for shipping instructions and special forms.

8–2). Anaerobic cultures should be transported promptly to the laboratory in a special anaerobic vial or in a syringe from which all the air has been removed and the needle stoppered.

Cultures of joint fluid are similar to culturing blood or secretions. It is important to perform cultures even if the Gram stain is negative; they are companion studies and not mutually exclusive.

Neisseria gonorrhoeae is fastidious, and infected joint fluid will colonize organisms only about one third of the time.[4] Best results are obtained by having chocolate agar, or for a potentially contaminated specimen, chocolate agar with three antibiotics (Thayer-Martin) culture plates at the bedside at 37° C. Immediately upon inoculation, place under 10% carbon dioxide (CO_2) and promptly return the plates to the laboratory for continued incubation for 2 to 10 days.

Culturing for fungi, acid-fast organisms, and viruses is also handled in standard fashion with growth patterns similar to that of blood cultures. It is highly advisable to alert the microbiology staff before arthrocentesis if special cultures are desired, so that preparations can be made ahead of time.

OTHER TESTS FOR INFECTION

Newer methods for rapid detection of septic arthritis are under clinical investigation. Gas-liquid chromatography reveals that elevated lactic acid levels in the range of 215 mg/dl are found in septic synovia as compared with 27 mg/dl in inflammatory arthritis and 23 mg/dl in noninflammatory arthritis. This test is of value even if antibiotic therapy has been started, and sequential data assist in evaluating response to treatment.[4a,b] In gonococcal infection, however, the lactic acid level is not high.[5] Additional peaks on the chromograph at 546 and 848 seconds consistent with *N*-valeric and *N*-hexanoic acid are present in gonococcal infection as well as other septic arthritis, but are absent in noninfectious states.[6] Succinic acid parallels lactic acid at lower concentrations, but succinic acid tends to stay elevated when lactic acid is normal in synovia aspirated after antibiotics have been administered. Diagnostically, neither of these short-chain fatty acids is more sensitive than a WBC count of greater than 50,000 mm³ or a glucose level of less than 40 mg/dl.[7] The test is expensive, but results are available in 4 hours. As gonococcal arthritis is the most common infection in adults, more sensitive tests are needed.

Countercurrent immunoelectrophoresis for microbacterial antigens also seems promising as a rapid (2-hour) test for specific organisms.[8] Fluorescent antibody techniques may also prove valuable.[9]

REFERENCES

1. Traycoff, R.B., Pascual, E., and Schumacher, H.R.: Mononuclear cells in human synovial fluid. Identification of lymphoblasts in rheumatoid arthritis. Arthritis Rheum., *19*:743, 1976.
2. Paul, H., Reginato, A.J., and Schumacher, H.R.: Alizarin red S staining as a screening test to detect calcium compounds in synovial fluid. Arthritis Rheum., *26*:191, 1983.
3. Shehan, H., and Storey, G.: An improved method for staining leukocyte granules with Sudan black. Br. J. Pathol. Bacteriol., *59*:336, 1947.
4. Manshady, B.M., Thompson, G.R., and Weiss, J.J.: Septic arthritis in a general hospital 1966–1977. J. Rheumatol., *7*:523, 1980.
4a. Behn, A.R., Mathews, J.A., and Phillips, I.: Lactate UV-system: a rapid method for diagnosis of septic arthritis. Ann. Rheum. Dis., *40*:489, 1981.
4b. Riordan, T., Doyle, D., and Tabaqchali, S.: Synovial fluid lactic acid measurement in the diagnosis and management of septic arthritis. J. Clin. Pathol., *35*:390, 1982.
5. Riley, T.V.: Synovial fluid lactic acid levels in septic arthritis. Pathology, *13*:69, 1981.
6. Brook, I., et al.: Abnormalities in synovial fluid of patients with septic arthritis detected by gas-liquid chromatography. Ann. Rheum. Dis., *39*:168, 1980.
7. Borenstein, D.G., Gibbs, C.A., and Jacobs, R.P.: Gas-liquid chromatographic analysis of synovial fluid. Arthritis Rheum., *25*:947, 1982.
8. Rytel, M.W.: Microbial antigen detection in infectious arthritis. Clin. Rheum. Dis., *4*:83, 1978.
9. Barr, J., and Danielsson, D.: Septic gonococcal dermatitis. Br. Med. J., *1*:482, 1971.

Chapter 9

Chemistry, Serology, and Immunology

ROUTINE CHEMISTRY

Table 9–1 shows normal and abnormal values for joint fluid chemical analyses. From a practical standpoint, most diagnoses are made on the basis of a good history and physical examination, gross and microscopic examination of joint fluid, Gram stain, and culture. Usually, chemical and immunologic studies offer only confirmative information at our present state of knowledge. Research in this area holds great promise, not only for clinical assistance, but also for illuminating basic pathogenic mechanisms of the rheumatic diseases.

Usually, synovia can be handled in the laboratory in the same fashion as serum. Occasionally, viscosity may be a problem; this can be remedied by dilution with normal saline solution or incubation with hyaluronidase. There are many variations on the incubation procedure. The one outlined is sufficient to remove all hyaluronic acid; if that is not necessary, then modify the procedure.

> Dissolve 3 mg of hyaluronidase powder per 1 ml of 0.15 N NaCl.
> Add 2 ml of resultant solution to 1 ml of joint fluid.
> Incubate this mixture at 37° C for 90 minutes.
> Dialyze the digestant against distilled water in the cold and remove the digested product.[1]

Table 9–1. *Joint Fluid Chemistry**

	Normal	Degenerative Joint Disease	Rheumatoid Arthritis	Infectious Arthritis	Ref.
Total Protein (g/dl)	2.1	2.99	4.19		42
Albumin (%)	56	57	42		
Alpha 1 (%)	8	6	8		
Alpha 2 (%)	7	8	11		
Beta (%)	11	12	14		
Gamma (%)	18	16	25		
Hyaluronic acid (mg/dl)	321	188	115	40	43
Cholesterol (mg/dl)	7.1	124	119		44
Phospholipids (mg/dl)	13.8	101	101		
Triglycerides (mg/dl)		65	50		

*See text for additional data.

Glucose

True glucose measurement of synovia as compared with blood at times helps to differentiate infection from inflammation; however, there is an overlap zone that decreases the test's value. Blood and joint fluid glucose should be obtained simultaneously after a fast of 8 hours. The degree of difference between the values of true glucose, being lower in the joint fluid, is the basis for the test. The Folin-Wu method of glucose determination is not specific and therefore not recommended. The autoanalyzer (ferricyanide) method is satisfactory, although it gives slightly higher results than true glucose by the glucose oxidase method, which is currently the optimal test.

In noninflammatory (normal) states, the differential between blood and joint fluid is less than 10 mg/dl; in inflammation, it may be up to 40 mg/dl. In infection, the differential is greater yet, but the area between 20 and 60 is an overlap zone depending on the intensity of the inflammation and/or infection. Certainly, when the absolute reading of synovial true glucose is below 20 mg/dl, infection should be strongly considered.[2] Rheumatoid arthritis activity of long standing in the involved joint may produce low glucose levels and represents the most difficult differentiation.[2]

Mucin Clot Test

This test correlates with the presence of inflammation as judged by WBC count and viscosity. Hyaluronate-protein (mucin), responsible for high viscosity, is a highly polymerized complex, which is apparently fragmented in the inflammatory process. The addition of acetic acid to joint fluid causes mucin to clot in the test tube. If inflammation is absent, there is no fragmentation of hyaluronate-protein, and a single firm clot forms. With inflammation, fragmentation occurs, and these fragments form many small clots. Usually, the test is unnecessary, but has great historical value.

The clot is either "good" (firm), "fair," or "poor" depending on how firm or friable is the clot (Fig. 9–1).

The original method of performing this supplementary test was described by Dr. Marion Ropes.[2] This method directs that one part whole joint fluid be added to four parts of 2% acetic acid and shaken. An alternative approach, if sufficient fluid is available, is to add a few drops of 2% acetic acid to the test tube containing synovia; watch the precipitate form as the acetic acid spirals down through the joint fluid. If clot potential is not obvious, then let settling occur for 1 to 5 minutes and then shake the tube. The result should be easily read. In the case of a turbid fluid, it is best to centrifuge the synovia and use the supernatant only.

Quantitative chemical determination of hyaluronate is available, which may be of special interest in research but is not necessary in clinical laboratory medicine.[1]

Proteins

The proteins in synovia are normally similar to those in plasma, but the relative amounts differ greatly. Albumin predominates. Fibrinogen, a larger molecule, is virtually absent, which accounts for the lack of normal clotting of even some hemorrhagic fluids. There is less total protein in synovia (2 g/dl) than in plasma. When inflammation appears, there is less molecular selectivity, and transudation of plasma components through the microvascular endo-

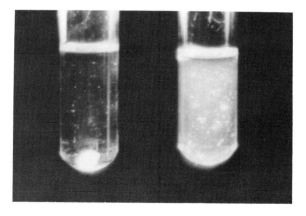

Fig. 9–1. Mucin clot; good (left), poor (right).

thelium causes joint fluid constituents, including proteins, to increase toward plasma levels.[3-5]

There is little clinical value in quantitating these individual proteins. Standard methods may be used, but hyaluronic acid must be removed first.

Lipids

Lipids (cholesterol, triglycerides, phospholipids, and neutral fats, like very low density lipoproteins) are present in synovia in low concentration, which increases with inflammation. Cholesterol in crystalline form has been discussed. Quantitation of lipids generally has no current clinical application, although fatty acid determination recently has been useful in linking lipolytic enzymes to the pathogenicity of arthropathy associated with pancreatitis.[6]

Urates

Uricase digestion of urate crystals initially was used to identify urate crystals in synovia. It has been replaced by the more specific methods and is mentioned only for historical value.[7] There is no value clinically in measuring total joint fluid urate as it mirrors serum values.

NEWER CHEMICAL STUDIES

A large number of investigations have been and are being performed. Some have promise and others may prove useful clinically; currently, they are of research value only. Awareness of this active research, however, adds a healthy perspective and optimism.

The lysozyme-to-lactoferrin ratio evaluates inflammation and cartilage degradation.[8]

Hydroxyproline levels are increased in crystal-induced arthropathies as compared with osteoarthritis and may be related to PMN interaction.[9]

Interferon,[10] ferritin,[11] fibrinectin,[12] collagenases,[13,14] platelet-derived connective tissue activating peptides,[15,16] arachidonic acid chemotaxis,[17] alpha-2 glycoprotein,[18] beta-2 microglobulin,[19,20] and collagen[21] have all been studied in joint fluid in relationship to inflammation and metabolism of cells and the synovial membrane.

ANTIBIOTICS

Evaluation of antibiotic concentration in joint fluid is performed as for serum. Multiple investigators have determined that, in the inflamed joint, high antibiotic levels are achieved.[22] Even during operations when a tourniquet is being used, intravenous antibiotics will pass through bone to the joint.[23] The clinical indication for measurement of antibiotic concentrations in joint fluid would be the uncommon case of septic arthritis that fails to respond to the appropriate antibiotic(s) in spite of serum levels well above the minimal inhibitory concentration.

SEROLOGY AND IMMUNOLOGY

In spite of the immense research effort in this area and the broad spectrum of information of great interest obtained, there is currently little value in performing these studies on synovia from a clinical diagnostic or prognostic standpoint. Hopefully, a breakthrough in clinical application will be forthcoming.

Rheumatoid factors are produced locally by synovial tissue cells and also appear in the serum. Therefore, on occasion, rheumatoid factors may be absent in blood, but present in low titer in the joint fluid.[24] This is still not disease specific, however, and does not warrant routine evaluation. Complement, although lower in joint fluid in rheumatoid disease and crystal-induced arthritis, is not of specific diagnostic assistance.[25,26] Immunologic studies of CIB,[27,28] analysis of immunoglobulins,[29] cryoprecipitins,[30] circulating immune complexes,[31-34] B-cells,[35] T-cells,[36] lymphocyte mobility,[37] antibodies (ANA, ADNA),[38] smooth muscle antibodies,[39] antigenicity of numerous constituents of joint fluid,[40,41] and many more are all areas of study that hopefully will have clinical application. New techniques of promise being used for these studies are C1q binding, Raji cell assay, radioimmune assay for circulating immune complexes, and rosette formation for lymphocyte subtyping.

REFERENCES

1. Cohen, A.S., Brandt, K.D., and Krey, P.K.: Synovial fluid. In *Laboratory Diagnostic Procedures in the Rheumatic Diseases*. Edited by A.S. Cohen. Boston, Little, Brown, 1975.
2. Ropes, M.W., and Bauer, W.: Synovial fluid changes in joint disease. Cambridge, Harvard University Press, 1953.
3. Kushner, I., and Somerville, J.: Permeability of human synovial membrane to plasma protein: relationship to molecular size and inflammation. Arthritis Rheum., *14*:560, 1971.
4. Pruzanski, W., et al.: Serum in synovial fluid proteins in rheumatoid arthritis and degenerative joint disease. Am. J. Med. Sci., *265*:483, 1973.

5. Levick, J.R.: Permeability of rheumatoid and normal human synovium to specific plasma proteins. Arthritis Rheum., *24*:1550, 1981.
6. Wilson, H.A., et al.: Pancreatitis with arthropathy and subcutaneous fat necrosis. Arthritis Rheum., *26*:121, 1983.
7. McCarty, D.J., and Hollander, J.L.: Identification of urate crystals in gouty synovial fluid. Ann. Intern. Med., *54*:452, 1961.
8. Bennett, R.M., and Skosey, J.L.: Lactoferrin and lysozyme levels in synovial fluid. Arthritis Rheum., *20*:84, 1977.
9. Manicourt, D., Rao, V.H., and Orloff, S.: Serum and synovial fluid hydroxyproline fractions in microcrystalline arthritis and osteoarthritis. Scand. J. Rheumatol., *8*:193, 1979.
10. Weinberger, A., and Pinkhas, J.: A hypothesis on the possible role of interferon in the initiation of acute gouty arthritis attack. Med. Hypotheses, *6*:781, 1980.
11. Blake, D.R., and Bacon, P.A.: Synovial fluid ferritin in rheumatoid arthritis: an index or cause of inflammation? Br. Med. J. (Clin. Res.), *282*:189, 1981.
12. Scott, D.L., Wainwright, A.C., Walton, K.W., and Williamson, N.: Significance of fibronectin in rheumatoid arthritis and osteoarthrosis. Ann. Rheum. Dis., *40*:142, 1981.
13. Giacomello, A., Salerno, C., Brundisini, B., and Fasella, P.: Collagenase activity in human synovial fluids from joint diseases of diverse etiology. Physiol. Chem. Phys., *12*:365, 1980.
14. Woolley, D.E.: Human collagenases: comparative and immunolocalization studies. CIBA Found. Symp., *75*:69, 1979.
15. Shapleigh, C., et al.: Platelet-activating activity in synovial fluids of patients with rheumatoid arthritis, juvenile rheumatoid arthritis, gout, and noninflammatory arthropathies. Arthritis Rheum., *23*:800, 1980.
16. Sloan, T.B., et al.: Connective tissue activation. XVI. Detection of a human platelet-derived connective tissue activating peptide in human sera and plasma and in synovial fluids and tissues. Proc. Soc. Exp. Biol. Med., *164*:267, 1980.
17. Klickstein, L.B., Shapleigh, C., and Goetzl, E.J.: Lipoxygenation of arachidonic acid as a source of polymorphonuclear leukocyte chemotactic factors in synovial fluid and tissue in rheumatoid arthritis and spondyloarthritis. J. Clin. Invest., *66*:1166, 1980.
18. Kasukawa, R., Ohara, M., Yoshida, H., and Yoshida, T.: Pregnancy-associated A2-glycoprotein in rheumatoid arthritis. Int. Arch. Allergy Appl. Immunol., *58*:67, 1979.
19. Todesco, S., et al.: Beta-2-microglobulin in synovial fluid of rheumatoid arthritis. J. Rheumatol., *7*:555, 1980.
20. Manicourt, D., Brauman, H., and Orloff, S.: Synovial fluid Beta-2 microglobulin and hydroxyproline fractions in rheumatoid arthritis and nonautoimmune arthropathies. Ann. Rheum. Dis., *39*:207, 1980.
21. Cheung, H.S., Ryan, L.M., Kozin, F., and McCarty, D.J.: Identification of collagen subtypes in synovial fluid sediments from arthritic patients. Am. J. Med., *68*:73, 1980.
22. Parker, R.H., and Schmid, F.R.: Antibacterial activity of synovial fluid during therapy of septic arthritis. Arthritis Rheum., *14*:96, 1971.
23. Schurman, D.J., Hirshman, H.P., and Burton, D.S.: Cephalothin and

cefamandole penetration into bone, synovial fluid and wound drainage fluid. J. Bone Joint Surg., *62*:981, 1980.

24. Rodnan, G.P., Eisenbeis, C.H., and Creighton, A.S.: The occurrence of rheumatoid factor in synovial fluid. Am. J. Med., *35*:182, 1963.

25. Kim, H.J., McCarty, D.J., Kozin, F., and Koethe, S.: Clinical significance of synovial fluid total hemolytic complement activity. J. Rheumatol., *7*:143, 1980.

26. McDuffie, F.C., and Clark, R.J.: Consumption of C3 via the classical and alternative complement pathways by sera and synovial fluids from patients with rheumatoid arthritis. J. Clin. Lab. Immunol., *2*:269, 1979.

27. Brandt, K., Cathcart, E.S., and Cohen, A.J.: Studies of immune deposits in synovial membranes and corresponding synovial fluids. J. Lab. Clin. Med., *72*:631, 1968.

28. Panush, R.S., Bianco, N.E., and Schur, P.H.: Serum in synovial fluid IgG, IgA, and IgM antigammaglobulins in rheumatoid arthritis. Arthritis Rheum., *14*:737, 1971.

29. Hasselbacher, P.: Extracellular aggregates of immunoglobulin in synovial fluid from rheumatoid arthritis. J. Rheumatol., *6*:374, 1979.

30. Ludivico, C.L., and Myers, A.R.: Survey of synovial fluid cryoprecipitates. Ann. Rheum. Dis., *39*:253, 1980.

31. Neoh, S.H., Bradley, J., and Milazzo, S.C.: Circulating and intra-articular immune complexes in rheumatoid arthritis: a comparative study of the C1Q binding and monoclonal rheumatoid factor assays. Ann. Rheum. Dis., *39*:438, 1980.

32. Male, D., Roitt, I.M., and Hay, F.C.: Analysis of immune complexes in synovial effusions of patients with rheumatoid arthritis. Clin. Exp. Immunol., *39*:297, 1980.

33. Hay, F.C., and Nineham, J.L.: Intra-articular and circulating immune complexes and antiglobulins (IgG and IgM) in rheumatoid arthritis: correlation with clinical features. Ann. Rheum. Dis., *38*:1, 1979.

34. Gupta, R.C., et al.: Comparison of three immunoassays for immune complexes in rheumatoid arthritis. Arthritis Rheum., *22*:433, 1979.

35. Konttinen, Y.T., et al.: Characterization of the immunocompetent cells of rheumatoid synovium from tissue sections and eluates. Arthritis Rheum., *24*:71, 1981.

36. Biberfeld, G., Nilsson, E., and Biberfeld, P.: T lymphocyte subpopulation in synovial fluid of patients with rheumatic disease. Arthritis Rheum., *22*:978, 1979.

37. Brown, K.A., Embling, P.H., Perry, J.D., and Holborow, E.J.: Electrophoretic behaviour of blood and synovial fluid lymphocytes in rheumatoid arthritis. Clin. Exp. Immunol., *36*:272, 1979.

38. Leon, S.A., et al.: DNA in the synovial fluid and the circulation of patients with arthritis. Arthritis Rheum., *24*:1142, 1981.

39. Mellbye, O.J., Fyrand, O., Brath, H.K., and Olsen, E.: Oligoclonal immunoglobulins and smooth muscle antibodies in arthritic joints. Clin. Exp. Immunol., *40*:103, 1980.

40. Alspaugh, M.A., Henle, G., Lennette, E.T., and Henle, W.: Elevated levels of antibodies to Epstein-Barr virus antigens in sera and synovial fluids of patients with rheumatoid arthritis. J. Clin. Invest., *67*:1134, 1981.

41. Ford, D.K., DaRoza, D.M., Shah, P., and Wenman, W.M.: Cell-me-

diated immune responses of synovial mononuclear cells in Reiter's syndrome against ureaplasmal and chlamydial antigens. J. Rheumatol., 7:751, 1980.

42. Decker, B., McKenzie, B.F., McGuckin, W.F., and Slocumb, C.H.: Comparative distribution of proteins and glycoproteins of serum and synovial fluid. Arthritis Rheum., 2:162, 1959.

43. Decker, B., McGuckin, W.F., McKenzie, B.F., and Slocumb, C.H.: Concentration of hyaluronic acid in synovial fluid. Clin. Chem., 5:465, 1959.

44. Cohen, A.S.: *Laboratory Diagnostic Procedures in the Rheumatic Diseases.* 2nd Edition. Boston, Little, Brown, 1975.

Chapter 10

Special Studies for Crystalline Material

The method of identification of pathologic crystalline structures in joint fluid under compensated polarized light microscopy has been described. These crystals and others are known to be present in joint fluid and soft tissue which, at times, cannot be as easily identified because of size or composition. In spite of this, they may be the inciting agent in an acute process. They are hydroxyapatite,[1-3] brushite,[4] whitlockite,[5] octacalcium phosphate,[6] calcium oxalate,[7] cryoglobulin,[8] lipid "liquid" crystals,[9] and possibly Charcot-Leyden crystals.[10]

Therefore, it is important to have a plan for processing crystal identification beyond optical methods with the polarizing microscope.

Stains are helpful, as noted in Table 8–1, and are simple to perform. They are not specific, however. Should further identification be necessary, the sophisticated equipment and skills of a reference laboratory will be required.

A brief description of available methods follows.

X-RAY DIFFRACTION

X-ray diffraction provides crystal lattice "d-spacings," which "fingerprint" crystals exactly on x-ray film in a pattern of arcs or rings. By comparing the d-spacings for placement and intensity of the unknown crystal with known crystals, exact identification, even

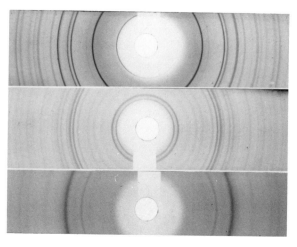

Fig. 10–1. X-ray diffraction powder patterns of dicalcium phosphate dihydrate (brushite), calcium pyrophosphate dihydrate, and hydroxyapatite (top to bottom). (From McCarty, D.J., Hogan, J.M., Gatter, R.A., and Grossman, B.S.: Studies on pathological calcifications in human cartilage. J. Bone Joint Surg., *48A*:309, 1966.)

down to the number of waters of hydration, can be made. Unfortunately, a minimum of 20 to 50 μg of crystals is needed for the standard microfocus instrument. This is quite a large amount to obtain from a single joint fluid, although easily obtainable from many soft tissue calcifications. Hydroxyapatite crystals can be identified by x-ray diffraction but are so small that fine definition requires electron microscopy (Fig. 10–1).

TRANSMISSION ELECTRON MICROSCOPY

Transmission electron microscopy, by focusing high-speed electrons onto an ultrathin specimen, then refocusing through electromagnetic lenses onto sensitive photographic film, can perform electron diffraction on a small specimen (2 to 3 Å or $10^{-10}M$), although the d-spacings are difficult to interpret with most routine transmission microscopes. This can be overcome in part by placing a known crystal on a split field with the unknown crystal and comparing the two resulting patterns visually for identity. This instrument also allows photography of crystals such as CPPD and hydroxyapatite that are not dissolved by the electron microscope fixatives (Fig. 10–2). With transmission electron microscopy, tiny crystals can be seen and their phagocytosis by various types of

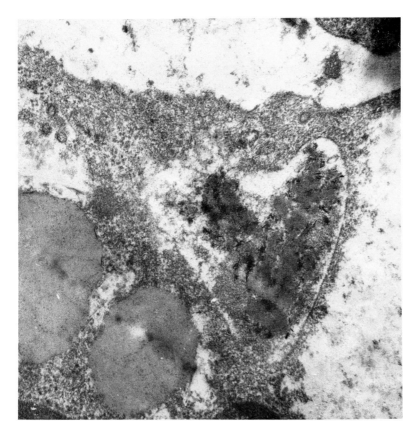

Fig. 10–2. Dark apatite needles in clump of protein-like material in joint fluid cell vacuole. Transmission electron microscopy. (Courtesy of H. Ralph Schumacher, M.D.)

cells can be documented. Investigative procedures such as use of peroxidase or ferritin conjugated antibodies to identify immunoglobulins on the surface of apatite crystals can be performed.

ELECTRON PROBE ANALYSIS

Electron probe analysis can identify the mineral content of crystals and allows calculation of the calcium-to-phosphate ratio of small quantities of the various calcium phosphate crystals under discussion (see the following).

SCANNING ELECTRON MICROSCOPY

Scanning electron microscopy can be used to analyze and photograph groups of whole crystals using a single drop of joint fluid with a three-dimensional image being created by light and dark shadows from the dispersion of reflected electron beams (Fig. 10–3).

These electron imaging instruments have helped define hydroxyapatite deposition disease and provided greater understanding of all the crystal-related disorders.[1,2,11–14] X-ray diffraction, likewise, has been a useful tool in defining each of the crystal-related disorders and pathologic calcifications in man.[3–7,15–18]

[14]CARBON-LABELED EHDP BINDING

[14]Carbon-labeled ethane-1-hydroxy-1-diphosphonate (EHDP) binding assay is used to confirm the presence of hydroxyapatite crystals as compared with CPPD. This test is sensitive to approximately 2 μg/mol of standard hydroxyapatite. Apatite will bind

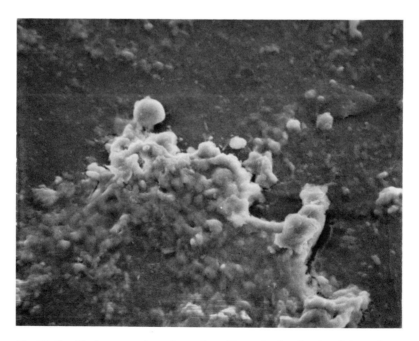

Fig. 10–3.   Hydroxyapatite microspheroids and other basic calcium phosphate crystalline material. Scanning electron microscopy ($\times 550$). (Courtesy of Paul B. Halverson, M.D.)

EHDP, whereas CPPD will not bind any. Other calcium phosphates such as octacalcium phosphate and carbonate apatite will also bind EHDP.[19]

INFRARED SPECTROPHOTOMETRY

Infrared spectrophotometry is used to analyze an unknown specimen for functional groups, e.g., phosphates. Also, a special form, Fourier transmission infrared analysis providing sequential electronic "stripping," gives in-depth analysis of these radials.[20]

CHEMICAL ANALYSIS

Chemical analysis for calcium:phosphate ratios of calcium phosphate crystals found in human tissues using standard methods are as follows:[21]

$Ca_5OH (PO_4)_3 H_2O$ (Hydroxyapatite) CA:P = 1.67
β-$Ca_3 (PO_4)_2$ (Beta tricalcium phosphate) (Whitlockite) Ca:P = 1.5
$Ca_8H_2 (PO_4)_6 5H_2O$ (octacalcium phosphate) Ca:P = 1.33
$CaHPO_4 2H_2O$ (dicalcium phosphate dihydrate) (Brushite) Ca:P = 1.0
$Ca_2 P_2 O_7 2H_2O$ (calcium pyrophosphate dihydrate) (CPPD) Ca:P = 1.0

FERROGRAPHY

Ferrography is a new approach to synovianalysis using magnetic trivalent Erbium to separate particles that become magnetized from those that do not take on a magnetic charge.[22] At present, it has no clinical applications, as it is only in the early stages of research evaluation.

CLINICAL APPROACH TO THE UNKNOWN CRYSTAL

It is best to discuss your needs with the reference laboratory, so that the most expedient method is used to obtain the desired result. Furthermore, not all of these tools will be available in a single reference laboratory. Established medical laboratories are listed in the appendix as starting points for such sophisticated analyses.

A typical case for investigation would be one with acute intermittent attacks of arthritis in one or a few joints revealing no crystals under compensated polarized light microscopy. Wright's stain reveals purple-staining clumps within PMNs, and alizarin red stain is positive for the same intracytoplasmic areas. This specimen would be sent for electron microscopic evaluation using transmission electron microscopy with electron diffraction for demonstration of crystals and for comparison with a known hydroxyapatite specimen.

A second typical case type would be acute or chronic arthritis with joint fluid or soft tissue crystals present that do not fit the definition of any known crystal. This specimen would be referred for x-ray diffraction.

REFERENCES

1. Schumacher, H.R., et al.: Hydroxyapatite-like crystals in synovial fluid cell vacuoles. Arthritis Rheum., *19*:281, 1976.
2. Dieppe, P.A., et al.: Apatite deposition disease. Lancet, *1*:266, 1976.
3. McCarty, D.J., and Gatter, R.A.: Recurrent acute inflammation associated with focal apatite crystal deposition. Arthritis Rheum., *9*:804, 1966.
4. McCarty, D.J., and Gatter, R.A.: Identification of calcium hydrogen phosphate dihydrate crystals in human fibrocartilage. Nature, *201*:391, 1963.
5. Gatter, R.A., and McCarty, D.J.: Pathological tissue calcification in man. Arch. Pathol., *84*:346, 1967.
6. Irby, R., Edwards, W.M., and Gatter, R.A.: Articular complications of homotransplantation and chronic renal hemodialysis. J. Rheumatol., *2*:91, 1975.
7. Hoffman, G.S., et al.: Calcium oxalate microcrystalline associated arthritis in end stage renal disease. Arthritis Rheum., *24*:73, 1981 (Abstract).
8. Langlands, D.R., et al.: Arthritis associated with a crystallizing cryoprecipitable IgG paraprotein. Am. J. Med., *68*:461, 1980.
9. Reginato, A.J., Schumacher, H.R., Allan, D., and Rabinowitz, J.L.: Acute monoarthritis associated with lipid liquid crystals. Arthritis Rheum., *25*:535, 1982 (Abstract 193).
10. Menard, H.A., deMedicis, R., Lussier, A., and Brown, J.: Charcot-Leyden crystals in synovial fluid. Arthritis Rheum., *24*:1591, 1981.
11. Schumacher, H.R., et al.: Acute gouty arthritis without urate crystals identified on initial examination of synovial fluid. Arthritis Rheum., *18*:603, 1975.
12. Honig, S., et al.: Crystal deposition disease, diagnosis by electron microscopy. Am. J. Med., *63*:161, 1977.
13. Faure, G., et al.: Scanning electron microscopic study of microcrystals implicated in human rheumatic disease. Scan. Electron Microsc., *3*:163, 1980.
14. Riddle, J.M., Bluhm, G.B., and Barnhart, M.I.: Ultrastructure study

of leukocytes and urates in gouty arthritis. Ann. Rheum. Dis., *26*:389, 1967.

15. Faires, J.S., and McCarty, D.J.: Acute arthritis in man and dog after synovial injection of sodium urate crystals. Lancet, 2:682, 1962.
16. Kohn, N.N., Hughes, R.E., McCarty, D.J., and Faires, J.S.: The significance of calcium phosphate crystals in the synovial fluid of arthritis patients: The pseudogout syndrome. II. Identification of crystals. Ann. Intern. Med., *56*:738, 1962.
17. McCarty, D.J., and Gatter, R.A.: Pseudogout syndrome. III. Articular calcifications—occurrence, distribution, and identity with crystals found in synovial fluid. Arthritis Rheum., *5*:652, 1962 (Abstract).
18. McCarty, D.J., Hogan, J.M., Gatter, R.A., and Grossman, M.: Studies on pathological calcification in human cartilage. I. Prevalence and types of crystal deposits in the menisci of 215 cadavers. J. Bone Joint Surg., *48*:309, 1966.
19. Halverson, P.B., and McCarty, D.J.: Identification of hydroxyapatite crystals in synovial fluid. Arthritis Rheum., *22*:389, 1979.
20. Halverson, P.B.: Personal communication.
21. *The Merck Index of Chemicals and Drugs.* Edited by Paul G. Strecher. 7th Edition. Rahway, N.J., Merck and Company, Inc., 1960.
22. Evans, C.H., et al.: Synovial fluid analysis by ferrography. J. Biochem. Biophys. Methods, 2:11, 1980.

Chapter 11

Clinical Significance of Joint Fluid Findings

Some clinical points have been touched on already in order to clarify certain areas. This chapter summarizes the general data that will help correlate the laboratory with the clinical aspects so that these findings are useful in the real world in which arthritis sufferers live.

Tables 1-1 and 1-2 provide the basic information relating joint fluid findings to clinical disease entities. The history, physical examination, blood studies, and roentgenograms will further clarify diagnoses. When crystals of MSUM and CPPD, bacteria, or definite neoplastic cells are proven to be in synovia, however, the diagnoses of gout, pseudogout, infection, or malignancy are established by definition.

Although "Group III" fluid is the "infectious" category, all categorization is artificial and exceptions should be expected. Low-virulence organisms, i.e., tuberculosis, gonorrhea, or partially treated infections may have Group II fluids. Conversely, inflammatory fluids are found with over 100,000 WBC per mm^3. Not uncommonly, more than one diagnosis is present. A septic process in a person with chondrocalcinosis can disrupt cartilage, dislodging CPPD crystals and causing secondary crystal-induced synovitis. This acutely painful, erythematous, and hot monoarthritis could pass for acute pseudogout alone if the differential diagnosis of septic joint were ignored once the crystals had been found on synovianalysis. Treatment could be local corticosteroid injection and discharge to home in the one instance, while hospital admission for parenteral antibiotics and joint drainage would be indicated in the other. There is no substitute for clinical acumen. The Gram stain must be done; the cultures must be taken in such cases.

Eosinophilia on differential WBC count suggests an allergic synovitis. This has been associated with arthrography,[1] chronic urticaria,[2] rheumatic fever,[3] parasitic infestation,[4] metastatic disease,[5] radiation therapy,[6] sclerosing injections for varicosities,[7] and rheumatoid arthritis.[8]

Monocytosis in synovia is seen with acute mononuclear arthritis and varicella arthritis.[9,10]

Lepra cells, foamy macrophages with intracellular degenerated lepra bacilli, which are Ziehl-Neelsen positive, have been reported.[11]

A predominance of lymphocytes has been found in rheumatoid arthritis in the first 6 weeks of disease activity, many of which are large "stimulated" cells.[12,13] These immunoblasts also have been found in Still's disease, psoriatic arthritis, and ankylosing spondylitis in greater numbers in the synovia than in simultaneous peripheral blood samples.[14,15] T-lymphocytes predominate in rheumatoid synovium.[16] Furthermore, T-lymphocytes counts are higher and B-lymphocytes lower in joint fluid than in peripheral blood in reactive arthritis.[17]

CIB are found more commonly in rheumatoid arthritis, but are nonspecific, are known to contain immunoglobulins and complement, and are not numerous in crystal-induced arthritis.[12,18,19]

Rice bodies are found in rheumatoid arthritis and juvenile rheumatoid arthritis. They are bits of fibrin-enriched degenerative synovium and its products and contain more Type B synovial lining cells than Type A, and about equal portions (40%) of Type I and Type III collagen with 20% Type V (A and B) collagen.[20–22]

Tumor cells seen on routine synovianalysis lead to cytologic study and more diagnostic testing for the origin of the neoplasm.[23]

The finding of grossly bloody synovia, lipid, or bone marrow spicules requires x-ray examination of the joint for fracture and clinical and laboratory evaluation for pancreatitis.[24–27] Blood alone in the joint may suggest a bleeding diathesis (see Table 1-2).

The presence of tubuloreticular structures or virus-like particles has been detected by electron microscopy in rheumatoid arthritis and other disorders; however, the significance of these findings is unknown at this time.[28]

Low complement and elevated immunoglobulins IgG, IgA, or IgM may be present in rheumatoid arthritis, systemic lupus erythematosus, and similar disorders. Recently, IgM cryoprecipitins in Lyme arthritis have been shown to correlate with disease activity.[29]

Crystal-induced arthritis was shown experimentally in dogs to be related to size of the crystal; e.g., diamond dust, which is amorphous, produced no synovitis.[30] Recent data seem convincing that, in spite of their size, sub(light)microscopic crystals, such as hydroxyapatite, can produce clinical synovitis.[31-33] Of great interest is the "Milwaukee Shoulder" syndrome, consisting clinically of destructive arthropathy, dislocation, absent rotator cuff, large noninflammatory effusion, and soft-tissue calcification. In this entity, hydroxyapatite crystals engulfed by synovial lining cells may stimulate these cells to produce neutral proteases and collagenase, which, in turn, break down articular cartilage and capsular fibrous connective tissue. It may be further speculated that articular cartilage degeneration may release crystals of various types (MSUM, CPPD, HA), which then theoretically might combine to produce a second inflammatory component to the joint disease.[34-36] The erosive arthropathies recently described in other joints associated with apatite crystals may be of similar etiology.[37]

Recurrent acute periarticular inflammation associated with apatite crystal deposition was described in 1966.[38] More recently, and with more sophisticated techniques, these crystals have been demonstrated in three clinical settings: acute calcific periarthritis, acute calcific arthritis, and in subacute to chronic arthritis resembling osteoarthritis.[33]

Hydroxyapatite is expected to be submicroscopic, but MSUM and CPPD can also be less than 1 μm.[39,40] This may account for some of the acute intermittent attacks of arthritis that occur without crystals being noted in joint fluid.

Other pathologic calcium crystals producing inflammation of joints and soft tissue are brushite,[41] octacalcium phosphate,[42] and calcium oxalate.[43] Whitlockite, although present in man, has not shown phlogistic properties to date. So far, renal failure and dialysis patients have exhibited calcium oxalate, calcite, and octacalcium phosphate crystals, although hydroxyapatite, MSUM, and CPPD also have been isolated commonly in these patients. Hydroxyapatite has been associated with octacalcium phosphate and, in one case, with tricalcium phosphate.[41]

CPPD is seen not only in large joints, but also in small joints, tendons, annulus fibrosus, tophaceous deposits, asymptomatic traumatic bunion joints,[44] the temporomandibular joint,[45,46] meniscal cysts,[47] and in a bursa.[48] Calcium pyrophosphate deposition disease is associated with several other findings, such as age (over 65), osteoarthritis, hyperparathyroidism, hemochromatosis, hemosiderosis, hypophosphatasia, hypomagnesemia, myxedema, gout, and amyloidosis.[49]

MSUM crystals not only can be aspirated from acutely inflamed joints with effusions, but have been found on aspiration of asymptomatic first metatarsophalangeal joints.[50]

Crystal deposition diseases may coexist with other forms of arthritis. In some cases, crystals cause secondary attacks with another primary inflammation or infection preceding them by several days; possibly, crystals are liberated by the enzymatic action that is taking place.

Cholesterol crystals are found in chronic effusions in joints and bursi, are not the cause of inflammation, and seem to have no relationship to systemic disease,[51] although, in animals, chronic synovitis has been induced by injection of cholesterol crystals.[52]

Slowly absorbed corticosteroid crystals injected into joints can produce postinjection "flares," including warmth, pain, and effusion with elevated white blood cell counts. The actual percentage of patients who have a symptomatic "flare" is not known, but it is small. Interestingly, some persons will develop transient high white counts and effusions without symptoms.[53] However, the clinical value of the injection is not diminished. Usually, an ice cap administered locally for 20 minutes is sufficient therapy for this self-limited complication. As mentioned earlier, prior to aspiration, it is important to know whether that joint had been injected in the past several months, as some crystals may still be present in the synovia on examination.

The presence of intracellular crystals means that they have been chemotactic for PMNs and, in turn, have activated the inflammatory process. Therefore, these crystals are a triggering agent for a pathologic event. In a given joint fluid, estimating and recording the percentage of intracellular and extracellular crystals is a gauge for how active the inflammation is on the basis of these crystals.

The mucin clot test was described earlier. It usually reflects the degree of inflammation present, being "poor" in the most inflamed fluid and "good" in the noninflammatory fluid. There are exceptions to this rule. Rheumatic fever and systemic lupus erythematosus may have a firm clot. Note, also, that these two diseases develop lower WBC counts at times than might be expected in a clinical setting of actively inflamed joints.

Synovianalyses for some of the less common disorders are noted in Table 11-1.

Table 11–1. *Joint Fluid Findings in Some Less Common Entities*

DISEASE	NUMBER OF PATIENTS	NUMBER OF FLUIDS	WBC/mm*	PMN%*	LYMPH%*	OTHER	REFERENCES†
Ankylosing spondylitis	6	12	7,000	46	38	Immunoglobulins higher, Lymphocytes lower, compared to RA	54
Sarcoidosis	1	1	14,800	24	74	RF 1:16‡ No crystals Mucin clot: firm	55
Fasciitis and eosinophilia	1	4	3,000	2	96	45% cells with CIBs	56
Milroy's disease	2	2	88	?	?	64% monocytes No crystals No cholesterol Mucin clot: good	57
Amyloidosis	5	11	3,300	variable		Large mononuclear cells No crystals High viscosity Amyloid fragments	58
Lipid inflammatory monoarthritis	4	6	24,000	89		Oil red O and Sudan Black + inclusions 1.5–2.0 μm Maltese cross inclusions under polarized light	59,60
Crystallizing IgG cryoparaprotein erosive arthritis	1	1	28,000	98		50 μm × 25 μm crystals, + and − elongation (Fig. 7–2)	61

*Represent averages.
†Not a complete list of references.
‡RF = rheumatoid factor.

REFERENCES

1. Hasselbacher, P., and Schumacher, H.R.: Synovial fluid eosinophilia following arthropathy. J. Rheumatol., *5*:173, 1978.
2. Klofkorn, R.W., and Lehman, T.J.A.: Eosinophilic synovial effusions complicating chronic urticaria and angioedema. Arthritis Rheum., *25*:708, 1982.
3. McEwen, C.: Cytologic studies on rheumatic fever. II. Cells of rheumatic exudates. J. Clin. Invest., *14*:190, 1935.
4. Bocanegra, T.S., et al.: Reactive arthritis induced by parasitic infestation. Ann. Intern. Med., *94*:207, 1981.
5. Goldenberg, D.L., Kelley, W., and Gibbons, R.B.: Metastatic adenocarcinoma of synovium presenting as acute arthritis. Arthritis Rheum., *18*:107, 1975.
6. Hasselbacher, P., and Schumacher, H.R.: Bilateral protrusio acetabuli following pelvic irradiation. J. Rheumatol., *4*:189, 1977.
7. Menard, H.A., deMedicis, R., Lussier, A., and Brown, J.: Charcot-Leyden crystals in synovial fluid. Arthritis Rheum., *24*:1591, 1981.
8. Panush, R.S., Franco, A.E., and Schur, P.H.: Rheumatoid arthritis associated with eosinophilia. Ann. Intern. Med., *75*:199, 1971.
9. Brawer, A.E., and Cathcart, E.S.: Acute monocytic arthritis. Arthritis Rheum., *22*:294, 1979.
10. Pascual, G.: Identification of large mononuclear cells in varicella arthritis (letter). Arthritis Rheum., *23*:519, 1980.
11. Louie, J.S., Koranski, J.R., and Cohen, A.H.: Lepra cells in synovial fluid of a patient with erythema nodosum leprosum. N. Engl. J. Med., *289*:1410, 1973.
12. Gatter, R.A., and Richmond, J.D.: Predominance of synovial fluid lymphocytes in early rheumatoid arthritis. J. Rheumatol., *2*:340, 1975.
13. Takasugi, K., and Hollingsworth, J.W.: Morphologic studies of mononuclear cells of human synovial fluid. Arthritis Rheum., *10*:495, 1967.
14. Eghtedari, A.A., Bacon, P.A., and Collins, A.: Immunoblasts in synovial fluid and blood in the rheumatic diseases. Ann. Rheum. Dis., *39*:318, 1980.
15. Traycoff, R.B., Pascual, E., and Schumacher, H.R.: Mononuclear cells in human synovial fluid. Identification of lymphoblasts in rheumatoid arthritis. Arthritis Rheum., *19*:743, 1976.
16. Ziff, M.: Relation of cellular infiltration of rheumatoid synovial membrane to its immune response. Arthritis Rheum., *17*:313, 1974.
17. Buelle, A.: Lymphocytes of synovial fluid and peripheral blood in reactive arthritis. A case report. Scand. J. Infect. Dis. (Suppl.), *24*:58, 1980.
18. Hollander, J.L., and McCarty, D.J.: Studies on the pathogenesis of rheumatoid joint fluid inflammation. I. The "RA cell" and a working hypothesis. Ann. Intern. Med., *62*:271, 1965.
19. Hannestadt, K.: Rheumatoid factor reacting with autologous native G globulin and joint fluid G aggregates. Clin. Exp. Immunol., *3*:671, 1968.
20. Wynne-Roberts, C.R., and Cassidy, J.T.: Juvenile rheumatoid arthritis with rice bodies: light and electron microscope studies. Ann. Rheum. Dis., *38*:8, 1979.
21. Cheung, H.S., Ryan, M., Kozin, F., and McCarty, D.J.: Synovial origins of rice bodies in joint fluid. Arthritis Rheum., *23*:72, 1980.

22. McCarty, D.J., Cheung, H.S.: Origin and significance of rice bodies in synovial fluid. Lancet, 715, Sept. 25, 1982.
23. Fam, A.G., Kolin, A., and Lewis, A.J.: Metastatic carcinomatous arthritis and carcinoma of the lung. A report of two cases diagnosed by synovial fluid cytology. J. Rheumatol., 7:98, 1980.
24. Lawrence, C., and Seife, B.: Bone marrow in joint fluid: a clue to fracture. Ann. Intern. Med., 74:740, 1971.
25. Berk, R.N.: Liquid fat in the knee joint after trauma. N. Engl. J. Med., 177:1411, 1967.
26. Graham, J., and Goldman, J.S.: Fat droplets and synovial fluid leukocytes in traumatic arthritis. Arthritis Rheum., 21:76, 1978.
27. Phillips, R.M.: Inflammatory arthritis and subcutaneous fat necrosis associated with acute and chronic pancreatitis. Arthritis Rheum., 22:355, 1980.
28. Schumacher, H.R.: Synovial membrane and fluid morphologic alterations in early rheumatoid arthritis: Microvascular injury and virus-like particles. Ann. N.Y. Acad. Sci., 256:39, 1975.
29. Steere, A.C., et al.: Lyme arthritis: correlation of serum and cryoglobulin IgM with activity and serum IgG with remission. Arthritis Rheum., 22:471, 1979.
30. McCarty, D.J., Gatter, R.A., and Pyenson, J.: Unpublished data, 1963-64.
31. Dieppe, P.A., Crocker, P., Huskisson, E.C., and Willoughby, D.A.: Apatite deposition disease: a new arthropathy. Lancet, 1:266, 1976.
32. Schumacher, H.R., Smolyo, A.P., Tse, R., and Maurer, K.: Arthritis associated with apatite crystals. Ann. Intern. Med., 87:411, 1977.
33. Fam, A.G., et al.: Apatite-associated arthropathy: a clinical study of 14 cases and of 2 patients with calcific bursitis. J. Rheumatol., 6:461, 1979.
34. McCarty, D.J., et al.: "Milwaukee Shoulder": Association of microspheroids containing hydroxyapatite crystals, active collagenase, and neutral protease with rotator cuff defects. I. Clinical aspects. Arthritis Rheum., 24:464, 1981.
35. Halverson, P.B., et al.: "Milwaukee Shoulder": Association of microspheroids containing hydroxyapatite crystals, active collagenase, and neutral protease with rotator cuff defects. II. Synovial fluid studies. Arthritis Rheum., 24:474, 1981.
36. Garancis, J.C., Cheung, H.S., Halverson, P.B., and McCarty, D.J.: "Milwaukee Shoulder": Association of microspheroids containing hydroxyapatite crystals, active collagenase, and neutral protease with rotator cuff defects. III. Morphologic and biochemical studies of an excised synovium showing chondromatosis. Arthritis Rheum., 24:484, 1981.
37. Schumacher, H.R., Miller, J.L., Ludivico, C., and Jessar, R.A.: Erosive arthritis associated with apatite crystal deposition. Arthritis Rheum., 24:31, 1981.
38. McCarty, D.J., and Gatter, R.A.: Recurrent acute inflammation associated with focal apatite crystal deposition. Arthritis Rheum., 9:804, 1966.
39. Buelle, H., Crocker, P., and Willoughby, D.: Ultra-microcrystals in

pyrophosphate arthropathy. Crystal identification and case report. Acta Med. Scand., *207*:89, 1980.

40. Honig, S., Gorevic, P., Hoffstein, S., and Weissman, G.: Crystal deposition disease: diagnosis by electron microscopy. Am. J. Med., *63*:161, 1977.

41. McCarty, D.J., and Gatter, R.A.: Identification of calcium hydrogen phosphate dihydrate crystals in human fibrocartilage. Nature, *201*:391, 1963.

42. Irby, R., Edwards, W.M., and Gatter, R.A.: Articular complications of homotransplantation and chronic renal hemodialysis. J. Rheumatol., *2*:91, 1975.

43. Hoffman, G.S., et al.: Calcium oxalate microcrystalline associated arthritis in end stage renal disease. Arthritis Rheum., *24*:73, 1981 (Abstract).

44. Dorwart, B.B.: Pseudogout crystals in asymptomatic toe joints. Presented, American Rheumatism Association, Southeastern Meeting. Charleston, S.C., December, 1980.

45. deVos, R.A., Kusen, G.J., and Becker, A.I.: Calcium phosphate dihydrate arthropathy of the temporomandibular joint. Oral Surg., *51*:497, 1981.

46. Pritzker, K.P., et al.: Pseudotumor of the temporomandibular joint: destructive calcium pyrophosphate dihydrate arthropathy. J. Rheumatol., *3*:70, 1976.

47. Good, A.E., Castor, C.W., and Weatherbee, L.: Pseudogout associated with meniscal cysts—report of two patients. J. Rheumatol., *5*:327, 1978.

48. Gerster, J., Lagier, R., and Boivin, G.: Olecranon bursitis related to calcium pyrophosphate dihydrate crystal deposition disease. Arthritis Rheum., *25*:989, 1982.

49. McCarty, D.J.: Crystal deposition diseases. In *Biennial Review of Rheumatic Disease.* Arthritis Foundation, Atlanta, 1982.

50. Weinberger, A., Schumacher, H.R., and Agudelo, C.: Urate crystals in asymptomatic metatarsophalangeal joints. Ann. Intern. Med., *91*:56, 1979.

51. Ettlinger, R.E., and Hunder, G.G.: Synovial effusions containing cholesterol crystals: report of 12 patients and review. Mayo Clin. Proc., *54*:366, 1979.

52. Pritzker, K.P., Fam, A.G., Omar, S.A., and Gertzbein, S.D.: Experimental cholesterol crystal arthropathy. J. Rheumatol., *8*:281, 1981.

53. McCarty, D.J., and Hogan, J.M.: Inflammatory reaction after intrasynovial infection of microcrystalline adenocorticosteroid esters. Arthritis Rheum., *7*:359, 1964.

54. Kendall, M.J., Farr, M., Meynell, M.J., and Hawkins, C.F.: Synovial fluid in ankylosing spondylitis. Ann. Rheum. Dis., *32*:487, 1973.

55. Varkey, B.: Synovial fluid in sarcoid arthritis. Ann. Intern. Med., *81*:557, 1974.

56. Rosenthal, J., and Benson, M.D.: Diffuse fasciitis and eosinophilia with symmetric polyarthritis. Ann. Intern. Med., *92*:507, 1980.

57. Frayha, R.A., Mooradian, A., and Khalid, F.T.: Transudative knee effusions in Milroy's disease. J. Rheumatol., *8*:670, 1981.

58. Gordon, D.A., Pruzanski, W., Ogryzlo, M.A., and Little, H.A.: Amy-

loid arthritis simulating rheumatoid disease in five patients with multiple myeloma. Am. J. Med., *55*:142, 1973.
59. Weinstein, J.: Synovial fluid leukocytosis associated with intracellular lipid inclusions. Arch. Intern. Med., *140*:560, 1980.
60. Reginato, A.J., Schumacher, H.R., Allan, D., and Rabinowitz, J.L.: Acute monoarthritis associated with lipid liquid crystals. Arthritis Rheum., *25*:535, 1982 (Abstract).
61. Langlands, D.R., et al.: Arthritis associated with a crystallizing cryoprecipitable IgG paraprotein. Am. J. Med., *68*:461, 1980.

Chapter 12

Technical Notes

COMPENSATED POLARIZED LIGHT MICROSCOPE

With the increased use of these microscopes, they have become increasingly available in the less expensive (nonresearch category) line of microscopes. Most major companies carry at least one such model. The price, which, of course, reflects quality and versatility, ranges from a few hundred to several thousand dollars. When looking for your first office microscope, work with a good outlet store or factory representative. If budget constraints are a factor, review the advantages of a reconditioned microscope with more comprehensive features. A new one with fewer features may serve you less well and cause you to trade it in sooner than anticipated.

Points for consideration are the following. First, there must be good optics throughout and easy adjustments for condenser and light source. Next, there must be a mechanical method of rotating crystals in relationship to the compensator while viewing the specimen without losing it from the microscopic field. The best method is a rotating microscope stage. Next best is a compensator that rotates 90° overlying the polarizer, which is on the base over the light source and a fixed stage (e.g., Leitz laborlux). This allows viewing of an individual crystal as though it had been rotated 90° to observe color changes. Not acceptable is an auxiliary mount for a fixed microscope stage, which rotates the wet preparation. It is not stable; thus, focus and/or field orientation are difficult to maintain. Finally, it is impossible to turn a wet preparation by hand on a fixed stage under higher powers. Remember that the demonstration slide offered by the sales representative usually contains multiple crystals oriented in all directions, making rotation seem unnecessary. An actual pathologic specimen, however, may have only one crystal in a high-power field, and rotation will be essential.

Check for stability of the entire microscopic system. Although adaptations can be used on a standard instrument, it is frustrating and difficult to analyze crystals if portions of the system are hand held and move erratically while the observer is looking through the eyepiece. A microscope adapted by the manufacturer is far superior, and this instrument can easily be used for ordinary light work by removing one polarizing disc.

Adapting an ordinary light microscope requires two polarizing discs, which can be obtained from your factory representative, cut from polarizing plastic sheets, or cut from the lens of polarizing sunglasses. The compensator can be produced by overlaying lengthwise two layers of transparent cellophane tape on a clean glass slide.[1] Be sure to test the taped slide with a known crystal slide, as tape thickness is critical to the colors transmitted. The polarizer, analyzer, and the compensator must be situated so that the wet preparation and compensator are between the polarizer and the analyzer. This system can work, but is not recommended.

Reversal of color under compensated polarized light is caused by reversal of image, which is an optical phenomenon. Reversal of image 180° is a common "built-in" artifact of most binocular microscopes, but does not alter the optical sign of a crystal. When certain beam-splitting teaching heads are used causing a mirror image to be projected through one or both heads, then crystal orientation will be altered 90° with respect to the compensator, but without change of color, causing misinterpretation of the optical sign.[2] Knowing this, a reference crystal can be used to determine if this error exists. If so, it is better not to ask the student to adjust his thinking, but rather to use a single head so that the technique learned can be transferred to other microscopes and to the literature.

Focusing problems have been dealt with earlier, in Chapter 6. In addition, there are several reasons why focusing under oil immersion becomes impossible without causing streaming of cells. These are inadvertent inversion of the slide with the cover slip down, two cover slips overlaid, elevation of one side of the slide off the stage surface by the mechanical slide holder, and a poor nail polish seal around the cover slip.

If your microscope is manufactured with all built-in features, then there is little need to standardize orientation of crystals beyond a first-time evaluation with a known crystal slide (a urate tophus is the best to use, as it has many needle-like crystals, is easy to obtain, and keeps well). For the adapted instrument that is reassembled before each use, it is wise to check a reference slide before each use while becoming familiar with your own system.

Most microscopes have one or more moving parts of the compensated polarizing system. For best results, slight adjustments should be made before viewing an unknown. After turning on the light source, adjust the polarizer and/or analyzer to provide the darkest field, which positions their axes mutually perpendicular, then adjust the compensator to give the brightest rose field, which should be at 45° to the axes of the polarizer and the analyzer.

COMPENSATED POLARIZED LIGHT AND CRYSTAL OPTICS[3]

Compensated polarized light differentiates optically positive (CPPD) from optically negative (MSUM) crystals by the *method of sensitive tints*. It is the change on rotation from blue to yellow or yellow to blue that defines optical signs as either positive or negative. Fortunately, the two most common crystals in acute arthritis have opposite optical signs. Plane-polarized light producing a dark field with bright white light crystals cannot provide this differentiation. The mechanism for differentiating positive from negative was outlined in the chapter on clinical application of this microscope. The optical reasons behind this result are of interest.

In general, compensated polarized light is an optical system whereby ordinary light is orientated into parallel planes; a portion of this light passes through a crystalline specimen to be examined and is altered by it; these alterations are magnified, and color is produced by the compensator. The emerging light is repolarized before reaching the eye. Figure 6–1 indicates the various segments of this process on the right and the composite light path on the left. In Diagram 1 in the right-hand column, incandescent (white) light passes upward through a polarizer, thus producing "plane" polarized light orientated in the direction of the arrow. All other light has been excluded. When a second identical polarizing plate (the analyzer), which has been rotated 90° to the polarizer, is placed in the light path, no light passes through it, and the microscopic field is totally dark.

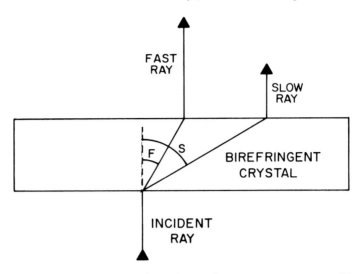

Fig. 12–1. Incident ray is refracted into divergent rays upon striking a birefringent crystal. (From Gatter, R.A.: Use of the compensated polarizing microscope. In *Crystal Induced Arthropathies*. Clinics in Rheumatic Diseases. Edited by William N. Kelley. Vol. 3. London, W.B. Saunders Co., 1977.)

Birefringence

In Diagram 2, a microscopic slide containing a MSUM crystal has been placed in the light path. This simulates the system inherent in a polarizing microscope without a compensator. The plane-polarized light, having been passed through the polarizer, strikes the birefringent urate crystals in the light path. Birefringence in this case means that the "incident" light, upon striking the crystal, is split into two refracted rays vibrating at different angles from the incident ray. The resultant ray with the greater angle of deviation from an optic axis will be slower passing through the crystal, and the ray with the lesser angle of bending will pass through more rapidly, thus producing a "slow ray" and a "fast ray" (Fig. 12–1). The vibration planes of these two new rays are mutually perpendicular, but neither are parallel to the original ray of plane-polarized light. Moreover, because of their different velocities, the slow ray and the fast ray are now out of phase with each other, as illustrated in Diagram 2. This emerging light is known as "elliptically" polarized light. As can be imagined, elliptically polarized light, being orientated differently from the original plane-polarized light, will have some portion capable of passing through the analyzer. The analyzer repolarizes the resultant rays, bringing to the eye the "bright" intensity of the birefringent sodium urate crystal superimposed on a dark field.

The Compensator

In Diagram 3, a compensator orientated 45° to the axes of the polarizer and the analyzer has been added to the system. This compensator is merely a more efficient birefringent structure. Note the arrow indicating its slow ray orientation (see left-hand column). Compensators are varied in thickness to transmit and retard various colors (light frequencies) of the spectrum and are named according to the light transmitted. They are usually made of quartz, mica, or gypsum. The birefringent quality of this material expressed numerically together with its thickness determines its characteristics expressed in nanometers. The clinical microscope is commonly fitted with a first-order red compensator, which is 540 to 575 nm. All the color changes referred to in this book relate to this one compensator.

A compensator has two important properties. First, it retards one of the colors of the spectrum of white light, a full wavelength,

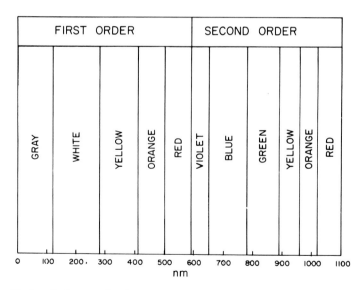

Fig. 12–2. Orders and colors in a polarized light system resulting from compensators theoretically from 0 to 1100 nm. (From Gatter, R.A.: Use of the compensated polarizing microscope. In *Crystal Induced Arthropathies.* Clinics in Rheumatic Diseases. Edited by William Kelley. Vol. 3. London, W.B. Saunders Co., 1977.)

thus essentially erasing it from the background illumination. In our case, green is eliminated, while red/orange/yellow and blue/violet are transmitted. Therefore, in Diagram 3, light reaching the eye reveals a background field which is no longer dark, but rose or "first-order red." Secondly, the compensator will produce interference colors, i.e., addition to the incident slow ray and subtraction from the incident fast ray, when each in turn is positioned parallel to the slow ray orientation of the compensator. For example, if either a CPPD or MSUM crystal were placed in the light path with its slow ray parallel to the slow ray of a first-order red compensator of 540 nm, the additive value would produce second-order blue (Fig. 12-2). If this same crystal were now rotated 90° so that its fast ray was parallel to the compensator's slow ray, a color subtraction of equal magnitude in nanometers would produce first-order yellow. Why? Because second-order blue and first-order yellow are approximately equidistant from first-order red (Fig. 12–2).

Elongation

One last determinant is needed to analyze crystals with this system. In the left-hand column of Figure 6–1, we see that the resultant image of the MSUM crystal is blue; therefore, from what has already been stated, the crystal's slow ray must be parallel to the compensator's slow ray orientation. Both MSUM and CPPD have this same characteristic, however. How then are they differentiated? By the relationship of their morphologic long dimension to their slow and fast rays. This is called elongation. By elongation, we can determine the crystal's optic sign as being either positive or negative (Fig. 12–3).

Both MSUM and CPPD crystals are biaxial. The two optic axes cross in an oblique fashion. For such crystals, the slow and fast rays bisect the angles formed by the optic axes. By definition, a crystal is optically positive (+) if the slow ray bisects the acute angles and negative (−) if the fast ray bisects the acute angles. Likewise, Figure 12-3 demonstrates that the morphologic long dimension of the physical crystal approximately parallels the ray that bisects the acute angle. The more narrow the crystal, the more true this statement becomes. Therefore, although we cannot see a light ray within a crystal, the sign of elongation can be determined by its color and relative physical position with respect to the compensator. This is easy to remember because it is logical. Slow ray parallel to slow ray (like rays) adds (+) color, i.e., first-order red up to second-order blue; compensator parallel to blue physical

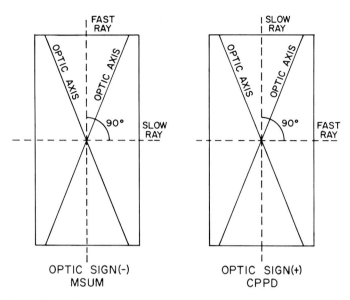

Fig. 12–3. Optical sign determination in biaxial crystals. The sign is positive (+) when the slow ray is the acute bisectrix of the optical axes and negative (−) when the fast ray is the acute bisectrix. (From Gatter, R.A.: Use of the compensated polarizing microscope. In *Crystal Induced Arthropathies.* Clinics in Rheumatic Diseases. Edited by William Kelley. Vol. 3. London, W.B. Saunders, 1977.)

crystal equals positive (+) elongation. The plus's (+) stay together. This is typical for CPPD. Slow ray parallel to fast ray (unlike rays) subtracts (−) color, i.e., first-order red down to first-order yellow; compensator parallel to yellow physical crystal = negative (−) elongation. Minus's (−) stay together. This is typical for MSUM and opposite from CPPD. It follows that if both crystals are rotated 90°, their other rays will be parallel to the compensator, and each crystal will change color from yellow to blue (MSUM) or from blue to yellow (CPPD), the physical crystals now being perpendicular to the compensator's slow ray.

Extinction

As noted previously, color changes related to optic axes, and the narrower the crystal, the more closely the optical axes are to the physical long axis. For example, MSUM changes colors crisply and is extinct on the exact plane of the polarizer and analyzer (Plate 4c). Broader crystals, such as CPPD, therefore, have less crisp changes fading gradually from one color to the next, with extinction occurring in an oblique relationship to the polarizer and analyzer.

This is true because the optic axes are obliquely placed within the crystal. "Oblique extinction" is the result.

Composite Light Path

Now we are ready to put this all together using the left-hand column of Figure 6–1. Here, in a composite of the compensated polarizing microscope, ordinary light first traverses the polarizer, whereupon it becomes plane polarized. Next it passes through the MSUM crystal and becomes elliptically polarized and enters the compensator. The MSUM crystal in this case is morphologically *perpendicular* to the slow ray orientation of the compensator (slow ray parallel to slow ray). The first-order red compensator imparts an additive blue interference color to the crystal, while at the same time retarding green, thus transmitting a resultant first-order red field. The elliptically polarized light passes, in part, through the analyzer and once again becomes plane polarized. The result is a blue crystal on a rose field.

CRYSTAL PHOTOGRAPHY

Assuming a proper photographic adaptation, camera, and alignment, photography can become a gratifying activity. Currently, Ektachrome 400 is a good basic film for wet preparations of crystals and for stained cells. Furthermore this film can be processed at 800 and 1600, thus decreasing the need for prolonged exposure times. This may change as advances in film sensitivity occur. Although exposure meters are available for this purpose, it is quite easy and more predictable to use time bracketing of exposures. Once familiar with your own results, bracketing one or two exposure settings on either side of your best exposure time should provide excellent photographs. Always use the same light intensity and condenser setting for consistent results. There may be some variation in quality relating to the amount of proteinaceous material present; if this is excessive, hyaluronidase pretreatment of the fluid will help provide clear images (see Chapter 9, "Routine Chemistry"). Note that image reversal can occur when focusing through the camera eyepiece, but the photograph will be as originally observed through the microscope eyepieces. It is wise to check focusing for sharpness periodically if long photography sessions of the same field are undertaken, as some shifting of cells may take place. Furthermore, if long exposure times are used, e.g., for fluorescent material, check for vibrations from other laboratory or building machinery. If such problems cannot be dampened sufficiently to obtain crisp images, then it may be necessary to do photography after regular hours when the offending equipment has been shut down. Special effects can be obtained by altering the condenser position so as to oblique the light slightly; phase objective and condenser are superior for this purpose.

STORING TEACHING MATERIALS

Joint fluid is best stored in test tubes in the refrigerator. The cellular structures will not remain intact, but crystals will. Slides can be kept for a short time, but they will dry out and be of little value. The exception to this is the urate tophus specimen that is essentially all crystalline material, and, therefore, dehydration has little effect on it.

REFERENCES

1. Owen, D.S. Jr.: Letter to the editor: a cheap and useful compensated polarizing microscope. N. Engl. J. Med., *285*:1152, 1971.
2. Nakonechny, D.S.: Image alerations in the teaching microscope. A source of error in synovial fluid crystal identification. Am. J. Clin. Pathol., *74*:392, 1980.
3. Gatter, R.A.: Use of the compensated polarizing microscope. In *Crystal Induced Arthropathies*. Clinics in Rheumatic Diseases. Edited by William Kelley. Vol. 3. London, W.B. Saunders, 1977.

Appendix I

Reference Laboratories for Unknown Crystal Identification

H. Ralph Schumacher, M.D.
Section of Rheumatology
Third Floor, Silverstein Building
Hospital of the University of Pennsylvania
Thirty-Fourth and Spruce Streets
Philadelphia, Pennsylvania 19104

Special interest: Electron microscopy.

Paul B. Halverson, M.D.
Rheumatology Laboratory, 5 East
Medical College of Wisconsin
8700 West Wisconsin Avenue
Milwaukee, Wisconsin 53226

Special interest: C^{14} EHDP binding and infrared analysis; scanning electron microscopy.

Neil Mandel, Ph.D.
Research Service/151
Veterans Administration Medical Center
Wood, Wisconsin 53193

Special interest: High-resolution x-ray powder diffraction.

Appendix II

Microscope Manufacturers and Distributors of Polarized Light Microscopes in the Northeast United States (partial listing)

American Optical Corporation
Scientific Instrument Division
Box 123
Buffalo, NY 14215

Bristoline Inc.
248 Buffalo Avenue
Freeport, NY 11520

Hacker Instruments, Inc.
Box 657
Fairfield, NJ 07006

New Jersey Scientific, Inc.
P.O. Box 165
Middlebush, NJ 08873

Olympus Corporation of America
4 Nevada Drive
New Hyde Park, NY 11042

Unitron Instrument Company
Microscope Sales Division
66 Needham Street
Newtown Highlands, MA 02161

Appendix III

Chemical Stains, Technique

ALCIAN BLUE METHOD (pH 2.5)

Fixation

10% neutral buffered formalin or Bouin's solution

Solutions

3% glacial acetic acid
Alcian blue staining solution
3% glacial acetic acid   100 ml
Alcian blue 8GX   1 g
Add a crystal of thymol to prevent mold growth.
Solution may be filtered back and reused. pH should be 2.5. Solution
is stable for about 2 months.
Nuclear fast red *(Kernechtrot)* counterstain or the PAS reaction may be
used.

Technique

1. Hydrate slides to distilled water.
2. Stain in the alcian blue solution for 30 minutes. Filter back.
3. Wash in running tap water for 2 minutes; rinse in distilled water.
4. Counterstain, if desired, with *Kernechtrot* for 3 to 5 minutes, followed
   by several changes of distilled water. Dehydrate, clear, and coverslip.
   Alternatively, the PAS reaction may be performed up to and including
   the 10-minute water wash after the sulfurous rinses. Dehydrate, clear,
   and coverslip, using a synthetic mounting medium.

Results

Carboxylated and sulfated acid mucosubstances and acidic mucins (with the exception of the strongly sulfated variety) are stained blue. With the *Kernechtrot* counterstain nuclei are colored pink-red and the cytoplasm is a pale pink. With the PAS counterstain, PAS-positive materials are colored magenta. Mixtures of both neutral and acidic mucosubstances are stained a purple color because of positive reactions with both the alcian blue stain and the PAS reaction.

ALCIAN BLUE STAIN (pH 1.0) FOR SULFATED MUCOSUBSTANCES

1. Hydrate sections.
2. Stain in 1% alcian blue 8GX in 0.1 N hydrochloric acid for 30 minutes. Filter back.
3. Rinse sections briefly in 0.1 N HCl.
4. Blot sections dry with fine filter paper. Do not wash in water, since this can change the pH and cause nonspecific staining to occur.
5. Counterstain, if desired. See preceding method, step 4. Otherwise, dehydrate, clear, and coverslip, using a synthetic mounting medium.

Results

Sulfated mucosubstances—blue

(Reprinted by permission of the publisher from "Specific staining of sulphate groups with alcian blue at low pH." by R. Lev and S.S. Spicer. J. Histochem. Cytochem., *12*:309, Copyright 1964 by Elsevier Science Publishing Co., Inc.)

ALIZARIN RED S STAINING AS A SCREENING TEST

One drop of fresh synovial fluid was mixed with one drop of 2% alizarin red S stain solution at pH 4.3 and then observed under regular and non-compensated polarized light within 3 minutes. This produced a heavy orange precipitate when calcium was present.

(Paul, H., and Reginato, A.: Alizarin red S staining as a screening test to detect calcium compounds in synovial fluid. ARA Abstracts, 23:730, 1980.)

MODIFIED CONGO RED STAIN OF BENNHOLD

Materials

Aqueous alum hematoxylin
Hematoxylin, 1 g
Saturated aqueous solution of ammonium alum, 100 ml
Distilled water, 300 ml
Thymol, a few crystals

Dissolve the hematoxylin in 300 ml. of distilled water by heating, add the thymol and ammonium alum, and expose the stain to the light in a bottle lightly stoppered with cotton until ripened. The stain is exposed for 30 days before use.

1% Congo red solution: 1 g of Congo red in 100 ml of 80% ethyl alcohol containing 0.1% NaOH

Polarizing microscope

Procedure

1. Stain sections of fixed or unfixed frozen tissue 10 minutes in 1% Congo red solution.
2. Wash in distilled water until clear.
3. Counterstain 10 to 15 seconds in aqueous alum hematoxylin.
4. Wash in running tap water until the sections are blue.
5. Dehydrate in 95% and 100% ethyl alcohol.
6. Clear in xylene and mount in Canada balsam or nonfluorescent mounting medium.

Results

In light microscope: amyloid, pink to red; nuclei, blue
In polarizing microscope: amyloid, green birefringence

(Cohen, A.S. (Ed.): *Laboratory Diagnostic Procedures in the Rheumatic Diseases.* 2nd Edition. Boston, Little, Brown, 1975.)

GRAM STAIN FOR SMEARS

1. Heat-fix air-dried smears.
2. Place on a staining rack and cover with a solution of crystal violet (1% aqueous, or Hucker's solution).
3. Drain off crystal violet and rinse with distilled water.
4. Cover slides with Gram's iodine and mordant for 30 seconds to 1 minute.
5. Drain off iodine and decolorize for 30 to 60 seconds with 95% ethanol, or for 5 to 10 seconds with acetone.
6. Wash with distilled water.
7. Counterstain 30 to 60 seconds in a 0.1% to 0.5% aqueous solution of safranin O.
8. Wash in distilled water, air-dry, and examine with oil immersion.

Results

Gram-positive organisms—blue to blue-black
Gram-negative organisms—red

(Reprinted by permission of the publisher from Lillie, R.D., and Fullmer, H.M.: *Histopathologic Technic and Practical Histochemistry.* 4th Edition. New York, McGraw-Hill, 1976.)

HEMATOXYLIN AND EOSIN

1. Hydrate slides
2. Suitably remove, if necessary, any mercury precipitate, formalin pigment, or yellow color caused by fixation in a picric acid-containing fixative such as Bouin's fluid.
3. Stain in *either* Delafield's, Ehrlich's, or Harris's formula for 8 to 15 minutes. (Experience will determine the best timing for a particular laboratory situation.)
4. Rinse slides in tap water to remove excess hematoxylin.
5. Differentiate using a 1% hydrochloric acid mixture in 70% ethanol. Usually 5 to 10 seconds is a sufficient time; however, this may have to be changed depending on the results of the subsequent microscopic examination.
6. Rinse well in tap water to remove excess differentiator; otherwise, the differentiating action will continue and result in a poor nuclear stain.
7. Blue the sections for 30 to 90 seconds in *either* a weak ammonia solution or a dilute lithium carbonate solution.

Ammonia solution

To 1 liter of tap water, add 3 ml of 28% ammonium hydroxide and mix.

Lithium carbonate solution

Equal parts mixture of filtered saturated aqueous lithium carbonate and distilled water.

8. Wash well in running tap water for 5 to 10 minutes. Inadequate washing after the bluing step will result in uneven eosin staining. Check microscopically. Sections should show blue nuclei with a well-defined chromatin pattern and nuclear membrane: cytoplasm should be almost colorless. *Note*: In some areas, prolonging the tap water rinse after bluing for more than 3 minutes can result in sections that are colored a brown-purple with poor nuclear detail.
9. Counterstain in the eosin solution of choice. Timing of the counterstain will vary from 15 seconds to 3 minutes depending on the freshness of the eosin solution and the depth of stain desired. Slight agitation of the slides may promote more even staining.
10. Dehydrate in two changes of 95% ethanol for 1 to 2 minutes each change. All excess eosin should be removed.
11. Dehydrate in two changes of absolute ethanol for 1 to 2 minutes each change.
12. Clear in an equal-parts mixture of absolute ethanol and xylene; follow this with two changes of xylene; coverslip using a synthetic mounting medium.

Results

Nuclei—blue
Cartilage and calcium deposits—dark blue
Cytoplasm and other tissue constituents—varying shades of red
Blood—bright red

(From Thompson, S.W., and Luna, L.G.: *An Atlas of Artifacts*, 1978. Courtesy of Charles C Thomas, Publisher, Springfield, Illinois.)

OIL RED O-ISOPROPANOL METHOD

Solutions

Stock solution
   Saturated solution of oil red O (300 mg/dl) in 99% isopropanol
Working solution
   Mix 6 parts of stock oil red O with 4 parts of distilled water. Allow to stand for 10 minutes. Filter this solution using Whatman no. 42 filter paper. Working solution is stable for 1 to 2 hours.
Ehrlich's or Harris's hematoxylin
0.05% aqueous lithium carbonate

Technique

1. Rinse sections in distilled water.
2. Stain in working solution oil red O for 6 to 15 minutes.
3. Clear background if necessary, using 60% isopropanol.
4. Wash well in distilled water.
5. Counterstain nuclei, using Ehrlich's hematoxylin for 2 minutes or Harris's hematoxylin for 30 seconds to 1 minute.
6. Rinse in tap water.
7. Blue sections in 0.05% lithium carbonate.
8. Rinse well in several changes of tap water or distilled water.
9. Coverslip, using an aqueous mounting medium.

Results

Lipids—red
Nuclei—blue

(From Lillie, R.D., and Ashburn, L.L.: Super saturated solutions of fat stains in dilute isopropanol for demonstration of acute fatty degenerations not showing by Herxheimer technique. Arch. Pathol., *36*:432, 1943. Copyright 1943, American Medical Association.)

GOMORI'S MODIFIED IRON STAIN (PRUSSIAN BLUE)

Solutions

10% potassium ferrocyanide
20% hydrochloric acid
Counterstain (*Kernechtrot*, eosin, etc.)

Method

1. Hydrate slides.
2. Immerse in 10% potassium ferrocyanide for 5 minutes.
3. Immerse in equal parts of potassium ferrocyanide and 20% hydrochloric acid for 30 minutes. Do not mix these two solutions together until just before use.

4. Wash thoroughly in distilled water.
5. Counterstain as desired (*Kernechtrot* for 5 minutes *or* 3% eosin for 30 seconds *or* 0.25% aqueous acid fuchsin for 20 seconds).
6. Rinse twice in distilled water.
7. Dehydrate, clear, and coverslip, using a synthetic mounting medium.

Results

Iron (ferric form)—bright blue
Background—depends on counterstain used

(From Gomori, G.: Microtechnical demonstration of iron. Am. J. Pathol., *12*:655, 1936.)

SUDAN BLACK B

(1) The dry film is fixed wih formaldehyde vapor by placing it for 5 to 10 minutes in a closed jar containing some 40% formalin in its lower part. This gives satisfactory fixation of erythrocytes as well as leukocytes.

(2) The Sudan staining solution should have a neutral or slightly alkaline reaction; if it is slightly acid, it stains only the granules of eosinophil leukocytes. It is improved by the addition of phenol, which appears to have a mordanting action on the granules.

Stock buffer solution. Sixteen g of crystalline phenol are dissolved in 30 ml of absolute alcohol. This is added to 100 ml of water in which 0.3 g of $Na_2HPO_4 \cdot 12H_2O$ has been dissolved.

Stock Sudan solution. 0.3 g of Sudan black B is dissolved in 100 ml of absolute alcohol. The dye must be completely dissolved. This can be ensured either by leaving the solution at room temperature for a day or two, with frequent shaking, or by grinding in a mortar and heating the resulting suspension.

For use, 40 ml of the buffer solution is well mixed with 60 ml of the Sudan solution and filtereed by suction. This buffered stain is ready for use at once; it can be used for several weeks, but becomes gradually slower in action with the lapse of time.

The fixed film is immersed in the buffered stain in a covered jar for 10 to 60 minutes. The longer times are required if the original stock Sudan solution was not completely dissolved or if the final stain is old or very cold.

(3) The slide is now well washed in absolute alcohol or 70% alcohol for a few minutes. The granules are only slowly decolorized by many hours' treatment with either absolute alcohol or xylol, though more quickly with acid alcohol.

(4) After washing in water, the slide is counterstained as desired. The most reliable stain is a 1:10 dilution of Gurr's Improved Giemsa R.66 in neutral water, allowed to act for 30 minutes. The blue tint of erythrocytes is then removed by differentiation for ½ to 1 minute in a 0.2% aqueous solution of KH_2PO_4. The film can be examined in immersion oil or can be mounted in balsam.

(From Shehan, H., and Storey, G.: An improved method of staining leukocyte granules with Sudan black. B.J. Pathol. Bacteriol., *59*:336, 1947.)

VON KOSSA SILVER TEST FOR CALCIUM

Fixation

Alcohol preferred; formalin may be used. Avoid calcium in the fixative solution.

Solution

5% aqueous silver nitrate solution
5% sodium thiosulfate
Nuclear fast red

Technic

1. Hydrate sections to distilled water.
2. Immerse slides in (or flood slides with) the 5% silver nitrate solution.
3. Expose the immersed (or flooded) slide to bright sunlight or ultraviolet light for 10 to 20 minutes or to a 60-watt electric bulb at a range of 4 to 5 inches for 60 minutes. Stop exposure when calcium salts are black-brown.
4. Wash slides in several changes of distilled water.
5. Remove unreacted silver with 5% sodium thiosulfate for 2 minutes.
6. Counterstain for 3 to 5 minutes with nuclear fast red. Filter back.
7. Rinse slides well in several changes of distilled water.
8. Dehydrate, clear in xylene, and coverslip, using a synthetic mounting medium.

Results

Calcium salts—black to brown-black
Nuclei—red
Cytoplasm—pink
Note: Oxalate salts are usually believed to give a negative Von Kossa reaction.

(From McManus, J.F., and Mowry, R.W.: *Staining Methods: Histologic and Histochemical.* New York, Harper & Row, 1960.)

WRIGHT'S STAIN

Solutions

Wright's stain (commercial)
Buffer solution
Sodium phosphate, dibasic	0.3 g
Sodium phosphate, monobasic	0.7 g
Distilled water	100 ml

Method

1. Lay thin blood smears face up on a horizontal staining rack.
2. Cover smear with Wright's staining solution (about 15 drops).

3. Let sit for 1 minute and then add twice the volume of distilled water, or instead of water, a 1:6 dilution of the above buffer stock solution. You should see a metallic sheen on the solution before proceeding with step 4. Allow the water or buffer and dye mixture to remain on the slide for at least 2 minutes.
4. Drain off and rinse with diluted buffer or distilled water until the thinner portions of the film are pink.
5. Blot dry, and mount in synthetic mounting medium.

(Reprinted by permission of the publisher from Lillie, R.D., and Fullmer, H.M.: *Histopathologic Technic and Practical Histochemistry.* 4th Edition. New York, McGraw-Hill, 1976.)

ZIEHL-NEELSEN STAIN

Solutions

Carbol fuchsin solution
Basic fuchsin	0.5 g
Distilled water	50 ml
Absolute ethanol	5 ml
Melted phenol crystals	2.5 ml

Filter solution before use
Decolorizing solution
   1% hydrochloric acid in 70% ethanol
   or
   1% aqueous sulfuric acid solution
Working methylene blue counterstain

Technique

1. Hydrate sections to distilled water.
2. Carbol fuchsin solution, 1 hour at room temperature.
3. Decolorize sections until tissue appears pale pink using either of the decolorizing solutions listed above.
4. Wash for 5 to 10 minutes in running tap water.
5. Counterstain in working solution of methylene blue for a few seconds. For better control of the stain intensity, individual slides may be carried through a Coplin-jar sequence of counterstain, alcohols, and xylene.
6. 95% alcohol, 2 changes.
7. Absolute alcohol, 2 changes.
8. Xylene, 2 changes. Coverslip, using a synthetic mounting medium.

Results

Acid-fast bacilli—bright red
Background—blue

(From Sheehan, D.C., and Hrapchak, B.: *Theory and Practice of Histotechnology.* 2nd Edition. St. Louis, The C.V. Mosby Company, 1980.)

Index

Page numbers in *italics* refer to figures; page numbers followed by "t" refer to tables.

103

Joint Fluid Characteristics

	Normal	GROUP I (Noninflammatory)	GROUP II (Inflammatory)	GROUP III (Septic)
Volume (knee, in ml)	<3.5	<3.5	>3.5	>3.5
Viscosity	Very high	High*	Low	Variable
Color	Clear	Xanthrochromic	Xanthrochromic to opalescent	Variable with organisms
Clarity	Transparent	Transparent	Translucent, opaque at times	Opaque
Mucin clot	Firm	Firm	Friable	Friable
WBC/mm^3	200	200–2,000	2,000–100,000	>50,000† usually >100,000
PMN (%)	<25	<25	>50	>75†
Culture	Negative	Negative	Negative	Usually positive

*Rapid accumulation of fluid will lower viscosity.
†May be lower with partially treated or low-virulence organism.

Differential Diagnoses by Joint Fluid Groups*

GROUP I (Noninflammatory)	GROUP II (Inflammatory)	GROUP III (Septic)	GROUP IV (Hemorrhagic)
Osteoarthritis	Rheumatoid disease	Bacterial infections	Trauma with or without fracture
Traumatic arthritis	Crystal-induced synovitis		Charcot's arthropathy
Avascular necrosis	gout		Hemorrhagic diathesis
Internal derangement	pseudogout		anticoagulant therapy
Osteochondritis dissecans	hydroxyapatite		von Willebrand's
Osteochondromatosis	corticosteroid injection		Hemophilia
Charcot's arthropathy	Psoriatic arthritis		Scurvy
Subsiding inflammation	Reactive arthritis		Thrombocytopenia
Villonodular synovitis	Reiter's syndrome		Hemangioma
Hypertrophic pulmonary osteoar-thropathy	Regional enteritis		Tumor
Systemic lupus erythematosus†	Ulcerative colitis		pigmented villonodular synovitis
	Postileal bypass		synovioma